OCCUPATIONAL THERAPY ASSISTANT CAREER PROFILE

OCCUPATIONAL THERAPY ASSISTANT CAREER PROFILE

by

NAOMI SCHUBIN GREENBERG,
Ph.D., O.T.R., F.A.O.T.A.

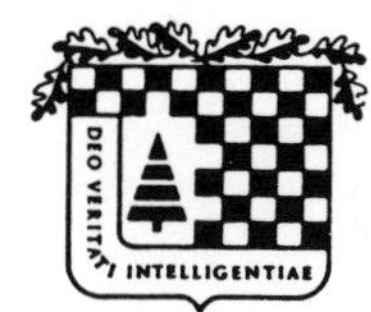

WARREN H. GREEN, INC.
St. Louis, Missouri, U.S.A.

Published by

WARREN H. GREEN
8356 Olive Boulevard
St. Louis, Missouri 63132, U.S.A.

ISBN No. 87527-270-3

Second printing, 1992
Third printing, 1997

Printed in the United States of America

Dedicated to

David, Seth and Ariel

in thanks for their dedication to me

INTRODUCTION

This book is designed for persons considering a career as an occupational therapy assistant, for health professionals and those in the community who wish to know about the role of the occupational therapy assistant and for beginning occupational therapy assistant students in an introductory course.

My original plan was to edit a text with each chapter written by a different occupational therapy assistant. But convincing occupational therapy assistants at that time to write rather than practice occupational therapy proved more difficult than I had anticipated. As this book evolved I maintained the concept of direct quotes from occupational therapy assistants, incorporating them into the chapters. Their positions as listed are as of the time the material was collected.

The book encompasses the broad spectrum of occupational therapy practice in the United States of America. It has been pretested in manuscript form and has enabled both potential and enrolled students to consider the appropriateness of occupational therapy assistant as a career choice. It serves to prepare the student for expectations in the field and provides an available reference for many questions which arise periodically throughout the training period. This work is based on country wide surveys, observations, interviews, and compilations of actual experiences of occupational therapy assistants in practice. In includes treatment examples of case studies reported by occupational therapy assistants based on their clinical encounters while actually on the job or in training for it. Hundreds of such reports were collected and culled for those which are most representative of the variety of experiences which occupational therapy assistants might encounter in their careers.

Occupational therapy is an evolving, growing field as is the health care delivery system in the U.S. in general. The role of the occupational therapy assistant is also evolving. It is for this reason that examples were not chosen from only the most traditional tasks and settings of the occupational therapy assistant but were selected to reflect the full scope of practice. It is fitting that this text is being released as the 30th anniversary of the Certified Occupational Therapy Assistant (COTA) is being celebrated.

Many people assisted in bringing this work to its completion. I wish to thank all those occupational therapy assistants who contributed by submitting information about their professional activities via letter, telephone and taped audio cassettes, and by responding to interviews and arranging for clinic observations. They are too numerous to list, but their experiences may be found among the pages of this book.

I also want to thank the directors and faculty of occupational therapy assistant schools for their suggestions, encouragement and referrals of occupational therapy assistants. The supportive efforts of present and former faculty, students and staff at LaGuardia Community College are also very much appreciated.

Thanks are also due to the staff of the American Occupational Therapy Association (AOTA) who provided appropriate data and relevant comments. AOTA documents and published materials are used with permission.

This book does not attempt to resolve the continuing dialogue of what the ideal role of the occupational therapy assistant should be. Nor is it meant to be all inclusive. Rather it enables the reader to glimpse what is happening in actual practice.

It is my hope that this compilation will foster recognition of the valuable contributions of the occupational therapy assistant and enable further growth in this significant health career.

Naomi Schubin Greenberg
December, 1989

TABLE OF CONTENTS

APPENDICES

OCCUPATIONAL THERAPY ASSISTANT CAREER PROFILE

PART I

OVERVIEW OF OCCUPATIONAL THERAPY AND THE OCCUPATIONAL THERAPY ASSISTANT

CHAPTER 1

IS OCCUPATIONAL THERAPY A NEW IDEA?

HISTORICAL PERSPECTIVES

Early History

The concept of involving patients in an activity in order to help them improve is not new. References to treatment by occupation are found in mythology as early as 600 B.C. Hippocrates, the father of medicine, in 200 A.D., emphasized the body-mind link suggesting exercise through riding, wrestling and labor. Galen, the Roman physician, directed treatment via such activities as digging, fishing and building.

More recent history involved early developments in the use of "invalid occupations" particularly in psychiatry. In 1906 Susan B. Tracy offered the first course in activities for the ill to nursing students and developed a manual called "Invalid Occupations." The students were presented with case studies, required to think of a suitable activity and make a sample. In 1913 Eleanor Clark Slagel, a hospital attendant, developed a program called "habit training," a daily program of scheduled activities in which self care was stressed. In 1918 Dr. William Dunton, a psychiatrist, formulated and published the first principles of occupational therapy. They reflected concepts that are still relevant today:

1. Activities should be directed toward a particular goal.
2. They should reflect the patient's interest.
3. Knowledge of the patient is important.
4. The activity should be changed or discontinued where indicated due to fatigue or other precautions.
5. Activities chosen should have a purpose.
6. The patient should gain knowledge or skill from the experience.
7. Interaction with others is important.
8. Encouragement and positive feedback should be provided.
9. The end product is not as important as the process.

George Barton is responsible for the name "occupational therapy" being used in 1914. He learned of its benefits as a result of his own illnesses which included tuberculosis, an amputated foot, and an emotionally based paralysis. He demonstrated through his own improved health that participating in activities (occupations) could help a person return to purposeful work.

The first conference to organize occupational therapy was held in 1917 at Consolation House in Clifton Springs, N.Y. which had been opened three years earlier by George Barton. He was elected president of the organization, and in 1916 chose the name, "The National Society for the Promotion of Occupational Therapy" (S.P.O.T.). A plaque commemorating the founding of what is now the American Occupational Therapy Association is located on the building at 16 Broad Street.

Highlights of the early history included the fact that by 1917 the organization had 40 members. In 1921 the name of the organization was changed to the American Occupational Therapy Association. By 1922 an official journal concerning itself with occupational therapy was initiated. In 1932 the first registry of occupational therapists was published and listed 318 names. A pledge and creed were adopted in 1926. The American Occupational Therapy Association, in 1933, was the first to initiate joint accreditation of health career training programs with the American Medical Association.

1935 brought the development of the "Essentials of an Acceptable School of Occupational Therapy." By 1945 occupational therapists were required to take a national examination after completing an accredited course in order to be registered occupational therapists. In 1947 the American Journal of Occupational Therapy began publication.

Creation of the Occupational Therapy Assistant Category

From just after World War II until 1958, persons who assisted occupational therapists were trained as occupational therapy aides through on the job training or short term courses. Since the American Occupational Therapy Association recognized the pressing need for new treatment personnel, the first AOTA approved occupational therapy assistant training programs were initiated. At first the programs were designed for specialty practice only. Many of the first training programs were located in large psychiatric facilities and focused heavily on teaching technical skills.

Then in the early 1960s, expanded occupational therapy assistant training programs were opened which included more theoretical material, provided more general foundations of the field and were 20–25 weeks long. In 1967 associate degree programs were introduced in community and junior colleges and by 1977 two-thirds of all new certified occupational therapy assistants were graduates of such programs. Nine to twelve month programs continued in some academic and clinical institutions.

Three stages in the history of national certification of the occupational therapy assistant took place. In the first stage were those who received certification based on previous supervised experience (grandfather clause) when approved programs and certification were first introduced. Over the next 20 years, graduates of approved training programs were deemed eligible for certification upon successful completion of an approved training program and recommendation of the program director. And finally in 1977, the first national examination was given as a prerequisite for certification and the use of the initials COTA. The development of state licensure for occupational therapy was occurring around the same time with Florida and New York enacting bills in 1975.

Recent Developments

In recent years the COTA has played an increasingly greater role within the national professional organization. An Award of Merit was granted to COTAs; the Roster of Honor designated a COTA for outstanding achievement each year; COTAs were elected to the representative assembly; a COTA advocacy position was established; a COTA Forum was introduced at annual conferences; a COTA Task Force was established, and a "COTA Share" column was created in "Occupational Therapy News." At the 1989 AOTA Conference a COTA received a unique honor as thousands celebrated the 30th anniversary of the COTA.

The 1980s also brought revised "Essentials for an Occupational Therapy Assistant Training Program" which require that such training be provided in a postsecondary educational institution (i.e., college or university level). A new patch to be worn on uniforms or other garments was designed for the COTA (Figure 1-1 shows the original patch). A new form for evaluation of occupational therapy assistant performance on fieldwork was approved and required. A COTA section of the official national occupational therapy newspaper was introduced. And recognizing the changing roles of occupational therapy personnel, the AOTA authorized the development of a new role delineation document. Table 1-1 lists highlights in the development of the COTA.

The future is bright for occupational therapy. The field and the occupational therapy assistant have come a long way since the early years. While both the profession and the first training programs for the occupational therapy assistant began in psychiatry or mental health, other areas of practice have surpassed it as occupational therapy moves into the 1990s and beyond.

IN THE WORDS OF AN OCCUPATIONAL THERAPY ASSISTANT

In order to understand who the COTA is and what the COTA is trained to do, let me take you through a journey to our past and clarify the profession's need to develop an assistant level.

During the 1940s, because of the countless numbers of war injuries, the profession was hard pressed to provide adequate personnel, not only to the Armed Forces, but also to the civilian hospitals and clinics. At that time, there were 6000 jobs available. But in 1949 there were only 375 graduates in occupational therapy. These numbers could not possibly meet the demand for occupational therapists nationwide. Therefore, The American Occupational Therapy Association (AOTA) education committee discussed the possibility of establishing a standardized hospital training program for assistants in psychiatric hospitals. In 1950, the education committee recommended further development of the plan, and proposed principles for the guidance of the Committee including:

1. That courses be given only under the supervision of an OTR;
2. That graduates of the program work only under the supervision of an OTR;
3. That consideration be given to some type of certification.

By 1951, in-service training for psychiatric aides had been carried out in several OT departments.

In 1953, the Board voted that a committee be appointed to make a study for proposed standards of training, accreditation, and recognition of non-registered personnel. And by June 1958, the State association presidents, and delegates received information concerning implementation of the plan. The guidelines charged among other things:

> That each training program should be set up to cover only one particular disability area and that the assistant be certified in that area.

The first AOTA approved program was offered by the Department of Mental Health at Westborough State Hospital in Massachusetts. The 12 week program became the pilot study to determine the effectiveness of established requirements.

In 1960—134 persons from 17 states had been certified. Yet, occupational therapy was like all other professions in the rehabilitation field, short of personnel. The OT consultants working in the area of physical disabilities stressed the need to recruit assistants. Requirements for an acceptable training program for assistants in general practice, procedures for certification of graduates of approved programs and a program outline were made available from AOTA. The last five years of the 60's and the first part of the 70's were mainly a period of learning, growth and adaptation. During that time, the COTA listing was established by AOTA, the AOTA by-laws were revised to include the COTA, and the first official guide for the supervision of the COTA was published in the American Journal of Occupational Therapy.

By 1982—25 programs had been approved in 17 states. All the programs used the same education essentials regardless of the length of time of each program. The minimal requirements for program content relating to occupational therapy were the same for the hospital based program, the one year academic program, and the associate degree program. In 1976, the AOTA developed the certification examination for COTAs to be used nationwide in order to assure that all COTAs have the same entry level body of knowledge. In 1978 the first Roles of Occupational Therapy Personnel was published by AOTA.

A task force was created which resulted in the appointment of a COTA advocate at the national level.

The 80s find COTAs faced with the challenge of new roles and new expectations and COTAs are beginning to become increasingly involved with American Occupational Therapy Association activities.

Angela Peralta, COTA

Excerpts from "Historical Background of the COTA" presented at the American Occupational Therapy Conference in Philadelphia in 1982.

SUGGESTIONS

1. Compare developments in occupational therapy and the occupational therapy assistant with events occurring historically at the time.
2. Identify the events in the development of occupational therapy that seem most significant to you and reasons why they appear to be more important.
3. Consider how a new health profession comes into being and whether events are similar for any new career area.

READING OBJECTIVES

1. Identify the area of practice first served by occupational therapy and the occupational therapy assistant.
2. Name the health career through which activities as therapy was first introduced.
3. Give examples of early use of occupational therapy approaches with patients.
4. State approximate years when the following occurred:
   Creation of an occupational therapy organization
   Approval of the first occupational therapy assistant training program
   Introduction of state licensure for occupational therapy
   The first national examination for the certification of occupational therapy assistants
   A new identifying "patch" for COTAs.

TABLE 1-1
HIGHLIGHTS IN THE HISTORY OF OCCUPATIONAL THERAPY AND THE OCCUPATIONAL THERAPY ASSISTANT

600 BC	References to treatment by occupation found in early mythology.
200 AD	Hippocrates suggested body-mind exercise through labor.
1906	Susan B. Tracy, a nurse, developed the first course and textbook entitled "Invalid Occupations."
1913	Eleanor Clark Slagel, a hospital attendant, developed a program called, "Habit Training," a daily program of scheduled activities in which self care was stressed.
1914	"Occupational Therapy," was named by psychiatrist, Dr. George Barton after experiencing its benefits through his own illness.
1917	The first conference to organize Occupational Therapy as a profession was held at Consolation House in Clifton Springs, NY (now historically recognized with a plaque).
1918	The first principles of Occupational Therapy were published by psychiatrist, Dr. William Dunton as reconstruction aides rehabilitated victims of World War I.
1921	The name of the professional organization became The American Occupational Therapy Association (AOTA).
1922	An official journal was initiated.
1947	The American Journal of Occupational Therapy (AJOT) began publication.
1959	First occupational therapy assistants certified.
1959	First AOTA approval granted to an occupational therapy assistant program.
1960	Requirements for an acceptable training program for occupational therapy assistants in general practice, procedures for certification of graduates of approved programs and a program outline prepared by AOTA.
1975	First Occupational Therapy State Licensure laws enacted.
1976	The first national certification examination was developed for occupational therapy assistants and used in 1977.
1978	The AOTA published "Roles of Occupational Therapy Personnel" comparing the registered occupational therapist (OTR) with the certified occupational therapy assistant (COTA).
1981	COTA Task Force created.
1984	New Essentials for the training of occupational therapy assistants require that programs be located in postsecondary educational institutions.
1985	New COTA identifying patch made available.

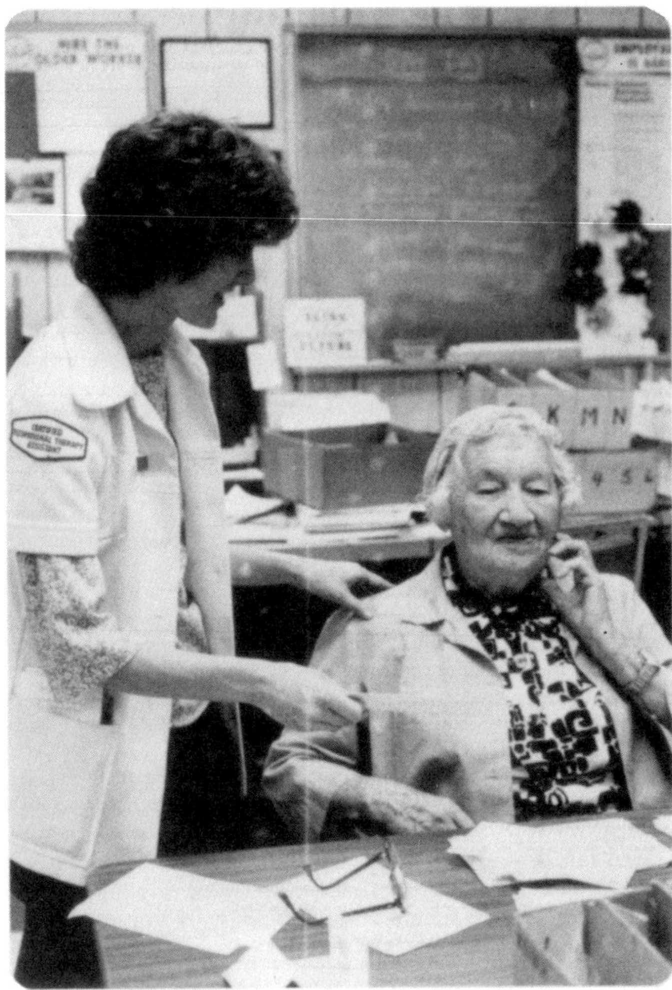

Figure 1-1: This photo showing an occupational therapy assistant in one of the newer roles of directing a paid workshop program for the aged, is now history. The Certified Occupational Therapy Assistant patch worn by the COTA was replaced by a new design in 1985.

CHAPTER 2

WHAT IS OCCUPATIONAL THERAPY?

OCCUPATIONAL THERAPY AS A CAREER

Definition

Occupational therapy, a growing specialty within the health care field, serves the needs of a variety of persons. It is a task oriented method used to help people to restore, reinforce and better their performance. It enables people to learn to deal with day-to-day situations which have become difficult as the result of deficiencies they were born with (i.e., physical malformations or mental retardation); age related changes in function; or physical or social impairment.

The main concerns of occupational therapy are to minimize those barriers (disabilities) which prevent the individual from functioning independently, as well as improve those factors (abilities) which help the individual to function. Thus a problem or concern is identified and an activity chosen to ameliorate it while enhancing the person's positive image and skills.

"Occupational" refers to occupied, busy, working, doing. Therapy refers to treating, helping or curing. Hence, "occupational therapy" may be thought of as treating by doing. Occupational therapy is practiced in many countries throughout the world. Thus, there are Portuguese, French, Hebrew, Hindustani, German, Italian, Greek, Japanese, Spanish and other equivalents to the term, usually translated from the English "healing through work." With increasing emphasis on licensure and individual states developing their own definitions of occupational therapy the following "Occupational therapy" definition for licensure was adopted.

> Occupational therapy is the use of purposeful activity with individuals who are limited by physical injury or illness, psychosocial dysfunction, developmental or learning disabilities, poverty and cultural differences or the aging process in order to maximize independence, prevent disability and maintain health. The practice encompasses evaluation, treatment and consultation. Specific occupational therapy services include: teaching daily living skills; developing perceptual-motor skills and sensory integrative functioning; developing play skills and prevocational and leisure capacities; designing, fabricating or applying selected orthotic and prosthetic or selective adaptive

> equipment; using specifically designed crafts and exercises to enhance functional performance; administering and interpreting tests such as manual muscle and range of motion; and adapting environments for the handicapped. These services are provided individually, in groups, or through social systems.[1]

The term, "purposeful activities" is the key to occupational therapy. In 1983 the Representative Assembly of the American Occupational Therapy Association (AOTA) adopted a position paper which stressed the importance of "purposeful activities" to the profession.[2] Excerpts follow:

> Occupational Therapists are committed to the use of purposeful activities. Purposeful activity is an important legitimate tool used by occupational therapists to evaluate, facilitate, restore, and maintain function.
>
> Individuals engage in purposeful activity as part of their daily life routine. Purposeful activity, in this natural context can be defined as tasks or experiences in which the person actively requires and elicits coordination between one's physical, emotional, and cognitive systems. Activities may yield immediate results or require sustained effort and multiple repetition.
>
> Occupational therapists treat individuals whose capacity to function effectively is impaired due to injury, illness, psychosocial stress, changing developmental and environmental demands, or lack of skill.
>
> Occupational therapy education in activity analysis and the behavioral and biological sciences provides the background necessary to use activities as therapeutic modalities for clients with a variety of physical, cognitive, emotional and social disorders.
>
> The activity is in itself an end, as well as being a means to a larger end.
>
> Occupational therapists divide activities into component parts to determine which skills are necessary to complete the task.
>
> Occupational therapists adapt activities in different ways to promote performance.
>
> Occupational therapists may present a series of activities, or change the steps within the activity. Such grading provide skill development and therapeutic exercise to respond to the dynamic changes of the client.
>
> Occupational therapists enable individuals to engage in purposeful activities to achieve competence in work, self-care, and play/leisure.
>
> Purposeful activities involve the doing processes which require the use of thought and energy and are directed towards an intended or desired end.

While Kathlyn Reed and Sharon Sanderson speak of occupational therapy as "the study of human occupations and the management of the adaptive behavior required to perform these occupational functions,"[3] Gary Kielhofner points out that "the simple theme defining occupational therapy in 1910 as the 'science of healing by occupations' still stands as the best reminder of what the occupational therapist is—an expert in the use of occupation as a health giving art."[4]

AOTA documents have described occupational therapy briefly as "the application of occupation or goal-directed activity to achieve optimum function, to prevent dysfunction, and to promote health."[5]

The official definition of occupational therapy remains:

> Occupational therapy is the art and science of directing man's participation in selected tasks to restore, reinforce and facilitate learning of those skills and functions essential for adaptation and productivity, diminish or correct pathology, and to promote and maintain health. Its fundamental concern is the capacity, throughout the life span, to perform with satisfaction to self and others those tasks and roles essential to productive living and to the mastery of self and the environment.[6]

Therapeutic Approaches

The occupational therapy assistant uses many approaches and techniques when carrying out direct service to patients or clients. Marie Louise Franciscus and Margarite Abbott[7] site specific activities used in occupational therapy, calling them "Tools of the Profession:" Creative and Manual Arts, Self-Help Devices, Orthotics, Prosthetics, Vocationally Related Activities, Energy Conservation Techniques, and Interpersonal Relationships.

Helen Hopkins and Helen Smith[8] speak of "Occupational Therapy Approaches for Intervention" in which they include:

Problem Solving Process
Development Approaches
Sensorimotor Approaches
Occupational Behavior Approach
Rehabilitation Approach

Within General Treatment Processes and Procedures they identify:

Therapeutic Adaptation of Activity
Activities of Daily Living and Homemaking
Prevocational Training
Biofeedback

Simme Cynkin states that "grouping activities under such headings as work-related, leisure time, social, recreational, and self-care reflects a view based on Western middle-class values and beliefs—of the categories to which activities properly belong and the relative importance attached to each. It soon becomes evident, however, that a number of specific activities fit quite appropriately into more than one category."[9]

In their definition of occupational therapy Kathlyn Reed and Sharon Sanderson include as "the means through which the results are achieved" the following: "analysis and training of daily living skills; design fabrication and application of orthotic and prosthetic devices; analysis, selection and use of adaptive equipment; selected application of sensorimotor, cognitive and psycho-social activities; use of therapeutically analyzed crafts, games and toys; task analysis and development of play, prevocational and avocational skills; and adaptation of physical environments (architectural barriers)." They index media as follows: avocational, creative arts, daily living tasks, exercise, functional equipment, manual skills, prevocation, recreation, use of self.

A regional survey of 500 clinical centers with regard to therapeutic activities for occupational therapy assistants[10] identified the following as key activities:

woodworking
activities of daily living
needlecrafts

Figure 2-1 shows the primary activity, woodworking, being used to meet a therapeutic goal. Woodworking is used by the occupational therapy assistant as a therapeutic activity in a variety of settings but also for the purpose of making or adapting equipment for special needs such as a wheelchair lap board. Two items made for the purpose of enhancing the activity of woodworking to meet therapeutic goals are an inclined sanding board with which the client can work against gravity to strengthen muscles, and a bilateral sander which can be weighted for resistance and which enables the client to use an unaffected arm to move an affected arm through its range of motion.

Woodworking is versatile. It can be used to meet mental health or cognitive goals, as an outlet for hostile feelings through hammering or sawing, or to give the client a sense of achievement through completing a project from start to finish. The latter promotes organizational skills, requires a sense of responsibility, and helps to build frustration tolerance.

Therapeutic approaches for the occupational therapy assistant may be grouped into five major areas: Activities of Daily Living (ADL), Therapeutic Activities, Therapeutic Exercise, Therapeutic Use of Self, and Pre-vocational Activities with additional specialty practices. These are listed in Table 2-2. More than one approach may be appropriately used to meet the occupational therapy goals for an individual along with "Therapeutic Use of Self." This refers to how the therapist or assistant is portrayed to the client including mannerisms, body language and facial expressions, words and tone used, and whether a response is quick or delayed. All may be designed for the therapeutic goal. A client may need to know for example that the occupational therapy assistant is firm or that the occupational therapy assistant is supportive.

Areas of Practice

Occupational therapy is now practiced with the "at risk" population as well as with those already identified as having a dysfunction. The former includes prevention programs, for example those which provide for infant stimulation among the socially or economically disadvantaged.

Areas of practice may be defined by age groups, e.g., geriatrics, or by dysfunction areas such as psychiatry or rehabilitation medicine, or by a broad area covering several concerns.

Developmental dysfunction is one such area. It is used currently to include a wide variety of conditions—developmental delay, learning disability, cerebral palsy, autism, mental retardation and some congenital deficits as well.

Six areas of practice of the occupational therapy assistant are highlighted in this book.

Three cover the major dysfunction areas of physical rehabilitation, developmental dysfunction, and mental health. Two are identified in terms of age groups—the aged and children. The remaining focuses on occupational therapy assistants in varied areas of practice which are less frequently experienced. There will be overlaps in roles and settings, for more than one area of practice may be found in the same setting—a general hospital for example. The collection is not meant to be all inclusive. There are many other types of patients and approaches in occupational therapy. Yet, a wide variety of roles are described for a general overview.

The functions of occupational therapy as defined by the American Occupational Therapy Association in its Definition and Functions[6] focus on three main types of programs within the areas of practice.

Prevention and Health Maintenance Programs are receiving increasing attention at this time and are a major focus of the occupational therapy assistant. This area includes activity programs as well as therapeutic approaches which enable a person to keep and use present abilities and to promote normal development.

Remedial Programs include rehabilitation—bringing the person back to a former level of functioning, and habilitation—bringing the person to a level not yet achieved.

Daily Life Tasks and Vocational Adjustment Programs focus primarily on the activities of daily living for a particular individual including exploration or readjustment of work related experiences which might include homemaking for the adult; play for the child; and tasks that prepare an individual for employment.

These areas are not exclusive. An individual's occupational therapy goals might cover all three. The same treatment modality or therapeutic approach may be directed to any one, two or three of the above.

Settings

Occupational therapy is practiced in a variety of settings both within institutions and the community. The most traditional location is the hospital setting. However, as hospital stays become shorter and community based health care programs become more prevalent, occupational therapy services are expanding into new settings in the community.

Hospitals may be general in nature or may specialize in areas such as psychiatry, chronic disease, or orthopedics. They provide the most intensive care with emphasis on the physician as the key member of the health care team.

Skilled nursing facilities (SNF) provide the next level of inpatient care with an emphasis on skilled nursing at the level of the registered nurse. Patients can be admitted to these facilities specifically for rehabilitation services of which occupational therapy is a part.

Health Related Facilities (HRF) are a less intensive form of residential care with a large amount of responsibility at the level of the practical nurse. Therapeutic communities and correctional facilities may also offer occupational therapy services as do some residences and group homes.

Community based services include day centers, community mental health centers, clinics, out-patient rehabilitation services, hand rehabilitation programs, schools, vocational workshops, and other types of settings. Services are also provided in individual clients homes.

Patricia Desler,[11] in stressing that changing health care patterns require more occupational therapy services in the community, emphasizes a need for a networking strategy to "deinstitutionalize the occupational therapist." The results she describes indicate that agencies which had never had occupational therapy services before are hiring COTAs into positions such as "skills trainer to work directly with patients placed in a semi-independent apartment program" and to provide socialization activities in centers.

Thus the settings in which occupational therapy assistants work are broadening, and may be determined by the need for occupational therapy services and the skills and knowledge of the occupational therapy assistant to meet that need. Table 2-3 provides a general list of settings.

IN THE WORDS OF AN OCCUPATIONAL THERAPY ASSISTANT STUDENT

In choosing a career, one has to know what the profession is about and one has to be interested and devoted to making that particular career enjoyable and rewarding. When a person is devoted to the occupation she or he has chosen, the rewards and levels of success will be well worth the hard work and dedication put into it.

Occupational therapy is just that profession for me. Helping people has always had its rewards, mostly through personal gratification.

Occupational therapy treats and trains patients who have physical, emotional and social deficits. It is a unique form of therapy in that it uses activity that is initiated by the patient and in which he actively participates. The occupational therapist trains a patient in the activities of daily living. The role of the therapist is vital in the community and to the rehabilitation of the patient.

The medical profession, as a whole, is a health team of which the occupational therapist has become an important member. He or she is there to help and will continue to be there serving and assisting the person who is deaf and blind, the physically and mentally disabled, the patient with tuberculosis or heart disease, children—whether they are physically handicapped or emotionally disturbed—and the senior citizen with arthritis or paralysis.

One can only summize the reward and feeling a trained therapist can receive when he administers aid and gives a sense of belonging to someone who can very easily be you or me.

Kenneth Barnes
Occupational Therapy Assistant Student

SUGGESTIONS

1. Find out where occupational therapy is provided in your community.
2. Visit one or more occupational therapy treatment programs.
3. Ask an occupational therapist and an occupational therapy assistant how they feel about their careers.
4. Be alert to occupational therapy being mentioned in newspapers, magazines, on the radio or television or in general conversations.
5. Talk to a recipient of occupational therapy services about the benefits of occupational therapy.

READING OBJECTIVES

1. Define occupational therapy in your own words.
2. State essential points in a definition of occupational therapy.
3. Discuss the meaning of "purposeful activities."
4. Explain how occupational therapy differs from other health professions.
5. Give examples of therapeutic approaches used by the occupational therapy assistant and the settings or areas of practice served.

REFERENCES

[1]AOTA: Handbook on Licensure, 1984.

[2]Hinajosa J, et al: Purposeful Activities. American Journal of Occupational Therapy 37:805–806, 1983.

[3]Reed K, Sanderson S: Concepts of Occupational Therapy. Williams and Wilkins, 1983.

[4]Kielhofner G: Occupation. Willard and Spackman's Occupational Therapy. Lippincott, 1983.

[5]American Occupational Therapy Association Recruitment Literature.

[6]American Occupational Therapy Association Council on Standards: Occupational Therapy: Its Definition and Functions, 1972 (Appendix I).

[7]Franciscus ML, Abbott M: Opportunities in Occupational Therapy. Vocational Guidance, 1979.

[8]Hopkins H, Smith H: Willard and Spackman's Occupational Therapy. Lippincott, 1983.

[9]Cynkin S: Occupational Therapy: Toward Health Through Activities. Little Brown, 1979.

[10]Early MB: "Survey of Therapeutic Activities for Occupational Therapy Assistants." Unpublished, 1985.

[11]Desler P: Deinstitutionalizing the Occupational Therapist. Occupational Therapy in Health Care. Spring, 1984.

TABLE 2-1
KEY POINTS IN A DEFINITION OF OCCUPATIONAL THERAPY

Types of persons treated:
- All ages
- Those with developmental, mental, physical or social limitations

Purpose:
- Enhancing or improving independent functioning for education, play/leisure, self care or work
- Preventing dysfunction
- Maintaining or promoting health

Means for achieving therapeutic goals:
- Purposeful activities
- Goal directed tasks

TABLE 2-2
THERAPEUTIC APPROACHES USED BY THE OCCUPATIONAL THERAPY ASSISTANT*

ACTIVITIES OF DAILY LIVING	THERAPEUTIC EXERCISE
Training in	Coordination
communicating	Range of motion
homemaking	Relaxation
dressing	Strengthening
grooming	Perceptual training
feeding	
transfers	THERAPEUTIC USE OF SELF
mobility	Encouragement
travel	Support
Assistive devices	Discipline
Adapted equipment	Structure
Energy conservation	Motivation
Time management	Role modeling
Architectural barrier modification	
	PRE-VOCATIONAL ACTIVITIES
THERAPEUTIC ACTIVITIES	Assembly tasks
Crafts	Clerical tasks
Games	Money management
Gardening	Packing
Music	Sorting
Cooking	Stacking
Dance and movement	
Current events	OTHER
Magic	Orthotic construction
Art	Prosthetic practice
Newsletter production	Sensory integrative follow through
Group Programming	Reality orientation
Discussion	Remotivation
Computers	Sensory training and stimulation
Community Activities	

*Independently, in collaboration with, or under the supervision of the occupational therapist.

TABLE 2-3
SETTINGS IN WHICH OCCUPATIONAL THERAPY IS PROVIDED

- Institutional
  - Hospitals
    - Psychiatric
    - General
    - Chronic disease
    - Specialty
  - Nursing homes
    - Skilled nursing facilities
    - Health related facilities
    - Intermediate care facilities
  - Correctional facilities
    - Forensic units
    - Detention centers
    - Security facilities
  - Other residential
    - Therapeutic communities
    - Group homes
    - Half way houses
    - Residences
    - Single room occupancy housing
  - Rehabilitation center
- Ambulatory Care (live out)
  - Clinics
    - Specialty
    - Rehabilitation
    - Hand
  - Community programs
    - Mental health centers
    - Day hospitals
    - Senior centers
    - Crisis intervention services
    - Independent living program
  - Other non-residential
    - Pain management clinics
    - Work evaluation
    - Sheltered workshops
    - Rehabilitation equipment suppliers
- Educational Sites
  - Schools
  - Learning centers
  - Developmental centers
  - Special education workshops
  - Infant stimulation programs
  - Pre-schoolers therapeutic play program
  - College teaching
- Home Care

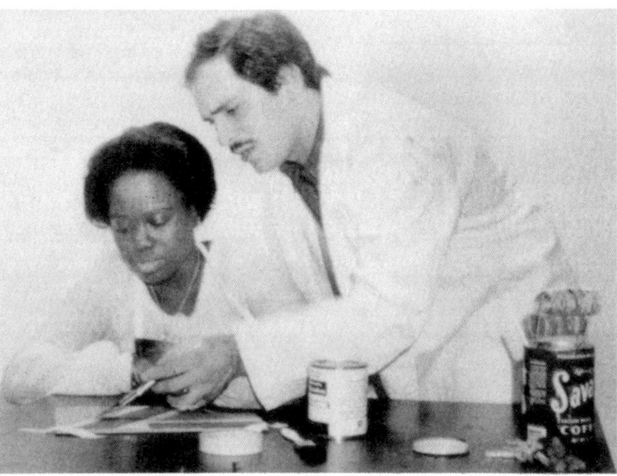

Figure 2-1: An occupational therapy assistant promotes decision making by demonstrating ways to choose a wood finish.

CHAPTER 3

WHO IS THE OCCUPATIONAL THERAPY ASSISTANT?

BEING AN OCCUPATIONAL THERAPY ASSISTANT

Description and Distribution

The occupational therapy assistant is a recognized member of the health care team who works independently or in collaboration with the occupational therapist in the delivery of occupational therapy services. Examples of responsibilities are shown in the job description which follows.

Although many individuals may assist in occupational therapy departments as explained in Chapter 5, the title occupational therapy assistant is being used to refer to the person who has completed an approved educational program for the occupational therapy assistant. Programs are approved by The American Occupational Therapy Association (AOTA) which also grants certification to graduates who successfully complete a national examination.

Certified Occupational Therapy Assistants may use the initials COTA after their names. Chapter 12 discusses certification.

The average age of COTA members of the American Occupational Therapy Association is 31 years, and more than three-fourths were trained at the associate degree level in occupational therapy. More than 20 percent of COTA's were pursuing additional degrees, as well.[12] Education and fieldwork requirements are covered in Chapter 4.

OCCUPATIONAL THERAPY ASSISTANT

Job Description *(from Dictionary of Occupational Titles)*

Assists occupational therapist in administering occupational therapy program in hospital, related facility, or community setting for physically, developmentally, or emotionally handicapped clients.

Assists in evaluation of clients' daily living skills and capacities to determine extent of abilities and limitations.

Assists in planning and implementing programs utilizing activities selected to restore, reinforce, and enhance task performances, diminish or correct pathology, and to promote and maintain health.

Designs and adapts equipment and working-living environment.

Fabricates splints.

Reports information and observations to supervisor.

Carries out general activity program for individuals or groups.

Assists in instructing patient and family in home programs as well as care and use of adaptive equipment.

Prepares work materials, assists in maintenance of equipment, and orders supplies.

May be responsible for maintaining observed information in client records.

There are many reasons why individuals choose the field of occupational therapy and specifically the role of the occupational therapy assistant. A Career Laddering study[13] identified the following six major reasons why students who were already in baccalaureate masters degree programs for the education of occupational therapists chose to apply to occupational therapy assistant programs:

Quicker entry into the field
Less investment in education
Increased emphasis on "doing" versus theory
Role preference
More supervision/less responsibility
More career versus liberal arts emphasis

One hundred such students transferred to occupational therapy assistant programs in the 5 year period ending 1982.[14]

The East, North Central, and Middle Atlantic areas of the country have the greatest concentration of occupational therapy assistants with the key states being New York, Minnesota and Wisconsin. These figures reflect locations where occupational therapy assistant training programs have existed over a long period of time. The Appendix shows the location of COTAs by state. In 1962, the first time membership figures for occupational therapy assistants were recorded, there were 761. By 1984 that number had grown to almost 7000 (nearly a 10 fold increase in 20 years) with representation in every state as well as the Virgin Islands and Puerto Rico. A survey of AOTA members abroad resulted in responses from COTAs in Canada, Israel, England and Germany. Forty percent of COTAs were licensed for practice in a particular state.

Clients Serviced and Functions

The types of practice of occupational therapy assistants may vary by state or region. A survey by the author through occupational therapy assistant educational programs showed great diversity regarding areas of practice of graduates. One OTA program reported only 10 percent of graduates working in nursing homes with the vast majority working in schools. Several other programs reported almost the opposite findings with geriatrics being a prime employment area for recent graduates.

Areas of practice also reflect nationwide trends. Tables 3-1 and 3-2 list the patient/client health problems most frequently encountered by occupational therapy assistants and the settings in which they are employed.

Frequent member data surveys by the American Occupational Therapy Association allow a comparison over the years and can indicate trends. In 1986 seventy percent of certified occupational therapy assistants (COTAs) responding to the survey were employed full-time. Six percent reported that they were self employed. The majority were working in private nonprofit institutions. Of 28 different practice settings on the survey form, categories listed most frequently were: skilled nursing home, school system, general hospital, psychiatric hospital and rehabilitation center. This reflects a new trend. School systems, which did not appear in the top categories 8 years previously grew to employ 14 percent of working COTAs. The vast majority of COTAs listed as their primary function "direct service" which included both evaluation and planning as well as implementation. On the average COTAs saw approximately 9 individual patients per day and conducted 3 group sessions. The primary health problems encountered by them were stroke (CVA/hemiplegia), mental retardation and psychosis. The highest categories of patient contact professional experience listed in a previous survey were self care performance (training patients/clients in activities of daily living) analysis, psychological functioning, social functioning and daily life adjustment. Program development was the key area of nonpatient contact experience. All ages were treated.

Table 3-3 shows primary experience areas of COTAs.

Professional Areas of Interest

A review of topics in which occupational therapy assistants expressed interest through the Hotline Column of the occupational therapy newspaper revealed the following:

Treatment approaches included movement and rhythm, community reentry, independent living programs, pre-vocational programs, activity programming, feeding and handwriting, mobility, play therapy, special chair programs, easy food recipes, personal computers, magic, sensory integrative process, motor skills, and tactile approaches. The problem settings or populations for which these would be used included learning disabled preschoolers, developmentally disabled adults, the retarded, rehabilitation clients, outpatient dialysis clients, half-way house residents, psychiatric patients, pulmonary rehabilitation patients, arthritic geriatric patients, cardiac care clients, clients with self-injurious behavior and autistic-like symptoms, pain management, home health programs, neurological patients, cystic fibrosis clients, physically disabled, private practice, head trauma patients, the elderly, multiple sclerosis clients, patients with Alzheimer's disease, the chemically dependent adolescent, the school system, the blind and visually impaired.

Table 3-4 lists specific areas of interest for which information was requested by COTAs.

IN THE WORDS OF AN OCCUPATIONAL THERAPY ASSISTANT

The COTA role was created by OTRs in response to a need for trained individuals who could carry out effective programs under supervision—providing health care for a larger number of patients. Today the success of programs may depend on the rapport established between OTR and COTA. The quality of the complementary or collaborative spirit can be the cohesive factor that accounts for a good program or an excellent one. COTAs could contribute to the documentation of research work. The role of the COTA is expanding and exciting careers are developing for and among today's COTAs. Brilliant role models include merit award winner Betty Cox, COTA, who served as Director of Communications for the AOTA and named to the Roster of Honor; Sally Ryan of the faculty of the College of St. Catherine, St. Paul, Minn., an Award of Merit winner and named to the Roster of Honor; Terry Brittell, appropriately chosen for the Award of Merit and named to the Roster of Honor for his devotion to patient care and loyal service to the New York State OT Association as an elected officer in several capacities. These are COTAs who have written and spoken about their work and are outstanding examples of the collaborative spirit between OTR and COTA.

The national association recommended utilizing COTAs in OTA educational settings. I had had five years experience as an Activities Director under the weekly supervision of an OTR consultant in a Home for the Aged before becoming an OT faculty member. I had graduated from a short term OTA program. Before that I had been illustrator of a "Do it Yourself" fashion column in the Sunday magazine section of the Philadelphia Inquirer and illustrator of a syndicated fashion column for the Chicago Sun Syndicate. At the same time I was married and by the time our fourth child was born I decided that the post-child period of my life should encompass something more meaningful than fashion. As time went on I became involved in Parent Teacher

Association and Girl Scouts. All these experiences contributed to my training in occupational therapy.

Choose the job in which you feel comfortable. Look for the supervisor who gives you a sense of dignity and relatedness. I can only wish you a future as rewarding and "expandable" as my own experience.

Gertrude Pinto, COTA[15]
New York State COTA of the Year

SUGGESTIONS

1. "Shadow" or observe an occupational therapy assistant in actual practice.
2. Think about the kind of job description you would want as an occupational therapy assistant.
3. Visit and compare two settings where occupational therapy assistants work.
4. Find out about some of the health problems that occupational therapy assistants treat.

READING OBJECTIVES

1. List examples of settings in which occupational therapy assistants are employed.
2. Name the health problems most frequently treated by occupational therapy assistants.
3. State reasons why an educational program for the occupational therapy assistant might be chosen over an educational program for the occupational therapist.
4. Identify tasks performed by an occupational therapy assistant.

REFERENCES

[12]American Occupational Therapy Association, 1986 Member Data Survey. September, 1987.

[13]American Occupational Therapy Association Commission of Education, Wisconsin Report on Career Laddering, 1984.

[14]American Occupational Therapy Association, Occupational Therapy Manpower: A Plan for Progress, 1985.

[15]Excerpts from "The Expanded Role of the COTA" presented at Erie Community College, 1981.

TABLE 3-1
MOST FREQUENT HEALTH PROBLEMS OF PATIENTS/CLIENTS

Health Problems	*OTRs %*	*COTAs %*
Acquired Immune Deficiency Syndrome (AIDS)	0.0	—
Amputation	0.2	0.3
Arteriosclerosis	0.3	0.6
Arthritis/Collagen Disorder	1.1	1.9
Back Injury	1.9	1.3
Burns	0.5	0.1
Cancer (Neoplasms)	0.3	0.3
Cerebral Palsy	11.7	7.9
Congenital Anomalies	0.3	0.3
CVA/Hemiplegia	28.2	27.6
Developmental Delay/Learning Disabilities	16.5	9.8
Diabetes	0.0	0.2
Eating Disorders	0.2	0.1
Feeding Disorders	0.2	0.2
Fracture	1.2	1.0
Hand Injury	7.2	2.0
Head Injury	3.3	2.6
Hearing Disability	0.1	0.3
Heart Disease	0.7	0.6
Kidney Disorder	0.1	0.1
Neuro/Muscular Disorder (e.g., MD, MS)	0.6	0.6
Respiratory Disease	0.2	0.1
Spinal Cord Injury	1.5	1.1
Visual Disability	0.3	0.3
Well Population	0.3	0.3
Adjustive Disorders	1.3	0.9
Affective Disorders	4.0	2.4
Alcohol/Substance Use Disorders	1.1	2.4
Anxiety Disorders	0.3	1.1
Mental Retardation	6.1	14.0
Organic Mental Disorders*	1.6	5.5
Personality Disorders	0.8	1.3
Schizophrenic Disorders	6.1	9.8
Other Psychotic Disorders	0.2	0.3
Other Mental Health Disorders	0.6	1.8
Other	0.9	1.0
Total	100.0	100.0

*Including Dementia, Alzheimer's and Organic Brain Syndromes.

Source: American Occupational Therapy Association 1986 Member Data Survey published September 1987.[12]

TABLE 3-2
PRIMARY EMPLOYMENT SETTING BY YEAR 1986

Setting	%
College, 2 year	0.8
College/University, 4 year	0.3
Community Mental Health Center	3.8
Correctional Institution	0.2
Day Care Center/Program	4.3
Halfway House	0.1
HMO (incl. PPO/IPA)	0.2
Home Health Agency	1.2
Hospice	0.0
General Hospital - Rehab.	4.5
General Hospital - all other	14.1
Pediatric Hospital	0.4
Psychiatric Hospital	8.4
Outpatient Clinic (free standing)	0.9
Physician's Office	0.2
Private Industry	0.5
Private Practice	1.9
Public Health Agency	0.4
Rehabilitation Hospital/Center	8.4
Research Facility	0.0
Residential Care Facility incl. Group Home, Ind. Liv. Ctr.	7.5
Retirement or Senior Center	1.1
School System (includes private school)	14.4
Sheltered Workshop	1.6
Skilled Nursing Home/Int. Care Facility	20.1
Vocational or Prevoc. Prog.	1.6
Voluntary Agency (e.g., Easter Seal/U.C.P.)	1.2
Other	2.2
Total	100.0

Source: 1986 Member Data Survey: Final Report, The American Occupational Therapy Association, September 1987.[12]

TABLE 3-3
EXPERIENCE-PROGRAMMATIC AREAS

Areas	%
Alcoholism & substance abuse	14.6
Architectural planning/design	2.1
Biomedical engineering	0.1
Cardiac rehabilitation	6.3
Driver training programs	0.2
Head injury programs	10.7
Neonatology	1.7
Orthotics	6.4
Pain management	2.9
Prosthetics	1.0
Seating & positioning	25.8
Sports injuries	0.8
Upper extremity injuries	18.1
Work programs (evaluation, hardening, worksite adjustment)	8.3
Work-related injuries	1.1
Total	100.0

Source: American Occupational Therapy Association 1986 Member Data Survey published September 1987.[12]

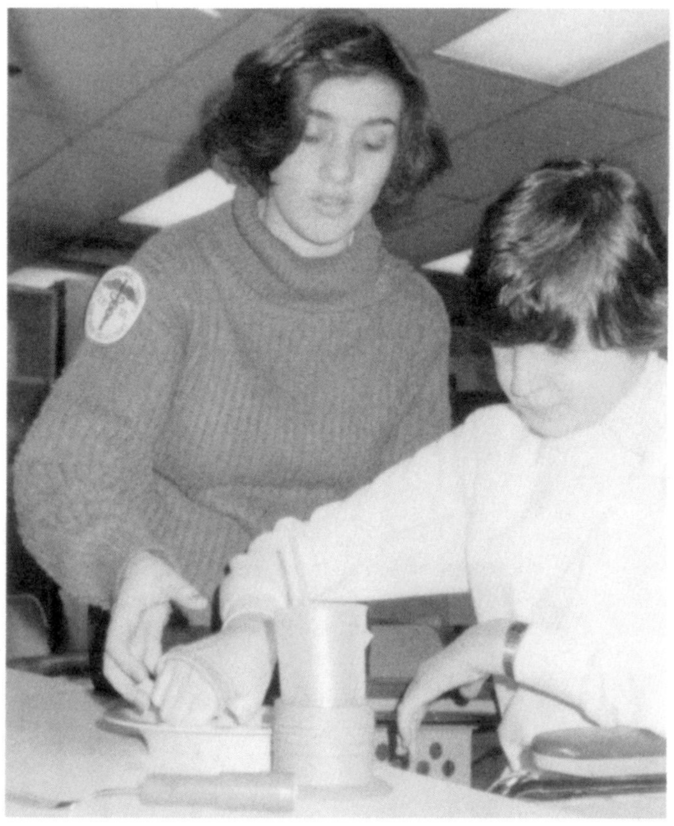

TABLE 3-4
EXAMPLES OF TOPICS OF INTEREST SUBMITTED BY COTA's TO THE AOTA HOTLINE COLUMN

- Movement and rhythmic form analysis for children
- COTAs in home health programs
- Community reentry programs with neurological patients
- Occupational therapy programs related to cystic fibrosis
- ADL dressing group in a physical dysfunction setting
- Occupational therapy assistants in cardiac rehabilitation
- Philosophical and practical career changes
- Independent living programs for physically disabled
- COTAs in private practice
- Pre-vocational program for handicapped and post head trauma patients
- Activity programming for patients with Alzheimer's disease
- Feeding and handwriting skills in multiple sclerosis patients
- Popular trends for OTs in the '80s working with the elderly
- OT with the chemical dependent adolescent
- Post CVA therapy group for an inpatient population
- Easy food recipes for chronically mentally ill, developmentally disabled, and physically disabled
- Programs for and parent involvement with visually impaired children ages infant through preschool
- Rocking Geri-chair
- Programs for learning disabled preschoolers
- Day service programming for developmentally disabled adults
- Modalities to control teeth grinding behavior in the retarded
- Prevocational evaluation forms for a rehabilitation setting
- Personal computers and software for patient treatment
- Project magic in any therapeutic setting
- Occupational therapy programs with outpatient dialysis patients
- ADL program for half-way house residents with recidivism
- The relationship of dysfunctional sensory integrative process to psychiatric patients
- Activities and mobility for the elderly blind/visually impaired
- Pediatric play therapy program
- COTAs working with dementia patients
- OTs working in any kind of holistic health care setting and the type of role they play
- COTAs working in employee assistance programs in public and private business

←

Figure 3-1: Enabling the patient to progress toward independence in eating is an important function of the occupational therapy assistant. Techniques such as guiding the hand through the proper movements may be used as well as a variety of assistive devices including built up handle utensils, suction holders, swivel spoons and plates with high sides.

CHAPTER 4

HOW IS THE OCCUPATIONAL THERAPY ASSISTANT EDUCATED?

EDUCATION OF OCCUPATIONAL THERAPY ASSISTANTS

Location of Programs

The American Occupational Therapy Association (AOTA) sets standards for and approves programs for the training of the Occupational Therapy Assistant. As of 1989 there were 65 such programs approved or pending approval in 32 different states throughout the country and in Puerto Rico. Table 4-1 and Figure 4-1 identify where programs are located.

Educational Content

Students must complete both an academic component of their education as well as a clinical or fieldwork component.

Although each school organizes its content differently, there are content essentials (Table 4-2) which must be included in the overall program in order for approval to be granted. The required content includes:

1. General Education
2. Biological, Behavioral, and Health Science
3. Occupational therapy concepts and skills
4. Values, Attitudes, and Behaviors
5. Fieldwork Education

Traditional training programs might organize content into theory courses and skills courses. One approach to theory content is a division by practice area, for example, one course on occupational therapy for physical dysfunction and a second on occupational therapy in the area of psychosocial dysfunction for children, adults, and the aged. A second approach offers three or four theory courses with separate courses on occupational therapy for the mentally retarded and/or the aged. Another approach uses a developmental concept with theory courses focusing on the child, the adolescent, the adult, and the aged with some age related areas grouped together. Generally the normal expected patterns of physical and psychological development are presented in separate courses before courses dealing with occupational therapy theory.

Skills courses include content on activities such as needlecrafts (Figure 4-2) and how they are used to meet therapeutic goals. They can be directed toward psychological benefits as diverse as promoting relaxation or building tolerance. Goals for physical rehabilitation include improving fine finger manipulation and maintaining range of motion (via the use of a long thread). Therapeutic aims important in any area of practice include color selection, matching size, and background discrimination.

Often two or three skills courses are offered with one or two focusing on craft techniques and their appropriate use in occupational therapy. As one example, needlecrafts are usually included as a means to teach (1) techniques needed to enable a patient or client to carry out specific steps and complete a project for therapeutic goals (such as fine finger coordination or cognitive skills) and, (2) techniques to enable the student to make therapeutic devices or adaptations such as a sling or a universal holder. Figure 4-2 shows one type of needlecraft.

At least one of the skills courses will introduce activities of daily living including techniques for training the patient or client in self care such as eating with limited mobility, transferring from a wheelchair to a bathtub or dressing with only one functional arm. Techniques for special populations as shown in Figure 4-3 or for energy saving approaches in the kitchen are usually included along with the use of assistive devices and the making of simple splints. Utilization of play or leisure activities is also included in skills courses as are pre-vocational exploration tasks such as assembling a ball point pen or nut and bolt set, or doing clerical work. Therapeutic use of self, communication and administrative content such as budgeting, ordering or managing an activities program are sometimes included in skills courses and other times found in separate modules.

One of the ways in which occupational therapy students learn techniques which they can in turn use to train their patients is by simulating a disability. For example, students may use a blindfold (Figure 4-3) to understand how a visually impaired person could find particular food on a plate if they are placed in accordance with the numbers of a clock, such as, "the peas are at the 3 o'clock position."

Likewise, content related to group leadership skills or to knowledge of the developmental aspects of potential clients or patients is sometimes found within occupational therapy courses themselves and other times designated to be covered within the framework of courses taught by another division of the educational institution. Examples of the latter might be "Sociology of Small Groups" or "Developmental Psychology." The advantage of keeping the required content within the occupational therapy courses is that it can be directed toward the specific population to be served and to the tasks of the occupational therapy assistant. However, by taking courses in other departments the student is exposed to a broader range of students, content and perspectives. This also allows for greater transferability of credits within the educational unit or upon transfer to another educational institution. Therefore, psychology, general biology or anatomy and physiology courses are usually included in the curriculum. Separate courses in pathology or medical and surgical conditions are also included in most cases.

High School Preparation

Many Occupational Therapy Assistant Education Programs do not have specific high school course requirements for admission. However, taking the following courses while still in high school is considered helpful: biology, English, mathematics. In addition courses in language and history or social studies are sometimes required to enter college or university programs with an approved major in Occupational Therapy. Some Occupational Therapy Assistant programs require minimum grades in overall or science courses. It is important that prospective students check with the selected college or university for its specific prerequisites for studying to be an occupational therapy assistant.

Educational programs for occupational therapy assistants are located in post secondary educational institutions. Most offer only day programs although three quarters accept part-time students. Evening and weekend options and individualized study programs exist.

AOTA data identify non-traditional options in occupational therapy assistant programs including: proficiency testing, life experience credit, acceptance of workshops or seminars, modifications of fieldwork. Figure 4-4 compares training for the occupational therapy assistant with training time for other health careers.

Students entering occupational therapy assistant programs generally fit into one of the following categories: recent high school graduates, transfer students, those seeking a second career, those seeking up-grading from a related position, and veterans or general equivalency diploma recipients.

Fieldwork Education

Over 2000 centers throughout the United States accept students for occupational therapy fieldwork. Each year approximately 900 occupational therapy assistant students complete both Level I introductory fieldwork and Level II advanced level fieldwork.

Level I Fieldwork requires patient contact during the academic program. Student observations during this experience help them to become aware of both the types of patients or clients who receive occupational therapy services as well as the types of settings and services offered. In most cases Level I fieldwork is built into a course as a separate block of time, but it might be scheduled as a separate course or components of several courses. Included in such experiences are field visits as well as scheduled assignments. Students could carry out such assignments on the basis of a half day per week throughout a semester for example, or even a full week during intersession. Level I fieldwork is sometimes referred to as a clerkship. Contracts or written agreements are signed by the educational institution with each affiliated fieldwork center for student placements for both Level I and Level II fieldwork.

Level II Fieldwork is traditional full-time experience often described as an internship or clinical placement. In order to be eligible for certification by the AOTA, every occupational therapy assistant must complete a minimum of two months of Level II fieldwork. Ideally this should include exposure to a variety of age groups, conditions and treatment approaches. To accomplish this many occupational therapy assistant programs place their students for two different Level II experiences and often extend the minimum requirement to 6 weeks or more in each of two different settings. Some programs require even more time as much as 8, or up to 13 weeks in each specialty area. In some cases students rotate to different clinics within the same setting.

Supervision is provided by an employee on site at the fieldwork center. An occupational therapist must plan and maintain responsibility for the fieldwork experience and is designated the fieldwork educator. The fieldwork educator can in turn designate another occupational therapist or occupational therapy assistant to provide direct supervision of the student. Supervision may be formal with scheduled meetings on a regular basis or informal with frequent contact between student and supervisor, or a combination of both. Supervision in occupational therapy means a two way interchange with both the student and the therapist raising questions, making suggestions and clarifying issues.

Objectives for the fieldwork experience are to be established in advance in conjunction with the occupational therapy assistant training program and are to be made known to the student. These objectives are discussed with the student during the first week of placement and reviewed periodically thereafter. It is suggested that a review of the student's progress be discussed at the mid-point of the placement period. Final evaluation of the student by the fieldwork educator or supervisor and of the center by the student are required. The student's performance is assessed in the areas of evaluation, treatment, communication and professional behavior. Table 4-3 identifies the specific areas in which the student is expected to perform. Once the student has successfully completed required fieldwork experience he or she is qualified for entry level practice.

Financial Considerations

The costs of completing an educational program for the occupational therapy assistant vary considerably throughout the country. Tuition is lower in government affiliated institutions. Some programs offer alternatives to traditional classroom courses for some segments of the curriculum. Thirty percent of all occupational therapy assistant programs offer scholarships specifically for occupational therapy assistant students. For all programs financial aid information is available. The American Occupational Therapy Association publishes a brochure on the subject and offers yearly scholarships. In addition, many state occupational therapy associations provide scholarships as do some government and voluntary health agencies and foundations.

In general, costs include tuition, student fees and textbooks. Some programs require uniforms. Liability insurance which is often required by the school to cover potential injury to a patient during student fieldwork is of relatively low cost. Students also need to plan ahead to cover the national certification examination fee and licensure fee if the student plans to work in a state which has occupational therapy licensure.

In most cases the clinical center does not receive payment for providing fieldwork supervision and education nor does the student receive reimbursement while completing the training experience. At present the cost of providing fieldwork placement opportunities is borne by the student, the center and the educational program. Students generally pay in one of three ways: tuition (the most frequent approach), placement fees, and special clinical fees. Stipends are sometimes provided for students during Level II placement. Stipends may cover uniforms, travel, lunches or a basic payment.

In *summary* the education of the occupational therapy assistant is based on standards established by the American Occupational Therapy Association. It includes a component in a clinical setting. Upon completion of an approved program, the occupational therapy assistant is eligible for the certifying examination.

IN THE WORDS OF AN OCCUPATIONAL THERAPY ASSISTANT

I decided to pursue a long time wish and become an occupational therapy assistant as a "second" career. I found the occupational therapy assistant training an excellent program of study—broad enough to allow for many areas of employment. I experienced excellent, warm support throughout my program. I had a B.A. degree, but going back to studying was challenging. Group dynamics, craft learning, progress note keeping, goal setting, knowledge of medical terms, medications, understanding effects of various disorders (physical and mental) and professionalism gave me confidence to apply for my current position.

As Coordinator of Adult Day Care it is my responsibility to make arrangements for attendance, transportation, programming, record keeping, raising money for special outings by craft sales, cooperating with the facility for space and shared activities and coordinating with health care workers for planning and progress regarding each participant. Participants come from their own homes and are provided with a hot meal, crafts, outings, exercise and interaction with other participants verbally and in games. Socialization is stressed, as many who come are isolated in their home environment. I have volunteers for staff; however, Activity Department staff in the personal care home make themselves available when needed, and we work very cooperatively.

Much is learned on the job, building on the OTA foundation.

A. Beverly Christianson, COTA
Coordinator of Adult Day Care
Convalescent Home of Winnipeg
Manitoba, Canada

SUGGESTIONS

1. Locate the occupational therapy assistant program nearest your home.
2. Learn the requirements for graduation from a selected occupational therapy assistant program.
3. Find out where occupational therapy fieldwork opportunities are available in your geographical area.
4. Talk with an occupational therapy assistant student or observe a class in session, if possible.

READING OBJECTIVES

1. Identify the required content of an occupational therapy assistant educational program.
2. State the requirements for fieldwork education for an occupational therapy assistant.
3. Name the college degree level that most occupational therapy assistant educational programs offer.
4. Compare the length of education required for an occupational therapy assistant with that of others in the health field.

TABLE 4-1
LOCATION OF EDUCATIONAL PROGRAMS* FOR THE OCCUPATIONAL THERAPY ASSISTANT AS OF 1988

Alabama	Kansas	North Dakota
California	Louisiana	Ohio
Colorado	Maryland	Oklahoma
Connecticut	Massachusetts	Oregon
Florida	Michigan	Pennsylvania
Georgia	Minnesota	Puerto Rico
Hawaii	Missouri	South Carolina
Illinois	New Hampshire	Tennessee
Indiana	New Jersey	Texas
Iowa	New York	Washington
	North Carolina	Wisconsin

*Approved or pending of approval by the American Occupational Therapy Association. The list published by the Association appears in Appendix.

TABLE 4-2
REQUIRED BASIC EDUCATIONAL CONTENT OF AN APPROVED OCCUPATIONAL THERAPY ASSISTANT PROGRAM

Content requirements shall include liberal and technical education.

1. General Education
   Prerequisite to or concurrent with technical education are those studies which include
   a. Oral and written communication skills.
   b. Socio-cultural similarities and differences.
2. Biological, Behavior, and Health Sciences
   a. Basic structure and function of the normal human body.
   b. Basic development of personality traits and learning skills.
   c. Environmental and community effects on the individual.
   d. Basic influences contributing to health.
   e. Disabling conditions commonly referred for occupational therapy.
3. Occupational therapy concepts and skills
   a. Human Performance
      Life tasks and roles as related to the developmental process from birth and death.
   b. Activity processes and skills
      (1) Performance of selected life tasks and activities, including self-care, work, play, and leisure.
      (2) Analysis and adaptation of activities.
      (3) Instruction of individuals and groups in selected life tasks and activities.
   c. Concepts related to occupational therapy practice including
      (1) The importance of human occupation as a health determinant.
      (2) The use of self, interpersonal, and communication skills.
   d. Use of occupational therapy concepts and skills
      (1) Data Collection
         Structured observation and interviews
         History
         Structured Tests

(2) Participation in planning and implementation
(a) Therapeutic intervention related to daily living skills and sensorimotor, cognitive, and psycho-social components.
(b) Therapeutic adaptation including methods of accomplishing daily life tasks, environmental adjustments, orthotics, and assistive devices and equipment.
(c) Health maintenance including mental health techniques, energy conservation, joint protection, body mechanics, and positioning.
(d) Prevention programs to foster age-appropriate balance of self-care, work, and play/leisure.
(3) Participation in Termination
Program termination including assisting in reevaluation summary of occupational therapy outcome, and appropriate recommendations to maximize treatment gains.
(4) Documentation
e. Participation in management of occupational therapy service
(1) Departmental operations: Scheduling, record keeping, safety, and maintenance of supplies and equipment.
(2) Personnel training and supervision: aides, volunteers, and level I OTA students.
(3) Data collection for quality assurance.
f. Direction of Activity Programs
(1) Assessment of individual needs, functional skills, and interests.
(2) Planning and implementation of programs to promote health, function and quality of life.
(3) Management of activity service.
4. Values, Attitudes, and Behaviors congruent with
a. The profession's standards and ethics.
b. Individual responsibility for continued learning.
c. Interdisciplinary and supervisory relationships within the administrative hierarchy.
d. Participation in the promotion of occupational therapy through professional organizations, governmental bodies, and human service organizations.
e. Understanding of the importance of occupational therapy research, publication, program evaluation, and documentation of services.
5. Fieldwork Education
a. Supervised fieldwork shall be an integral part of the technical education program.

Source: American Occupational Therapy Association, Essentials of an Approved Education Program for the Occupational Therapy Assistant, 1983.[18]

TABLE 4-3
AREAS OCCUPATIONAL THERAPY ASSISTANT STUDENTS EXPERIENCE DURING FIELDWORK*

1. Evaluation (ability to collect, use, and apply evaluative data)
   a. Use available sources for collecting evaluation data
   b. Select information from data sources
   c. Elicit pertinent data from interviews
   d. Obtain pertinent data from observation
   e. Correctly administer assigned evaluation procedures
2. Treatment/Program Planning and Treatment Implementation
   a. Develop a program based on short- and long-term goals.
   b. Carry out programs that reflect identified goals.
   c. Give instructions and select media and techniques
   d. Use the techniques of group process to achieve group goals.
   e. Identify and report the need for program change.
   f. Consider each client's needs and background when initiating and establishing a relationship.
   g. Attend to safety needs of client.
   h. Respond in a therapeutic manner to specific manifestations of client behavior.
3. Communication
   a. Orient client and client's family members to OT program.
   b. Communicate with supervisor to facilitate treatment goals.
   c. Communicate with relevant others regarding overall goals.
   d. Maintain accurate written records and reports.
4. Professional Behavior
   a. Budget time for preparation, cleanup, or review.
   b. Maintain equipment, supplies, and treatment area in good order.
   c. Take advantage of opportunities to learn new techniques.
   d. Modify behavior in response to supervisory feedback.
   e. Respect clients' rights to confidentiality, privacy and choice.
   f. Handle personal and professional problems so that they do not interfere with performance of duties.
   g. Adhere to policies and procedures of the facility.

*Based on AOTA Fieldwork Evaluation Form for Occupational Therapy Assistant Students.[20]

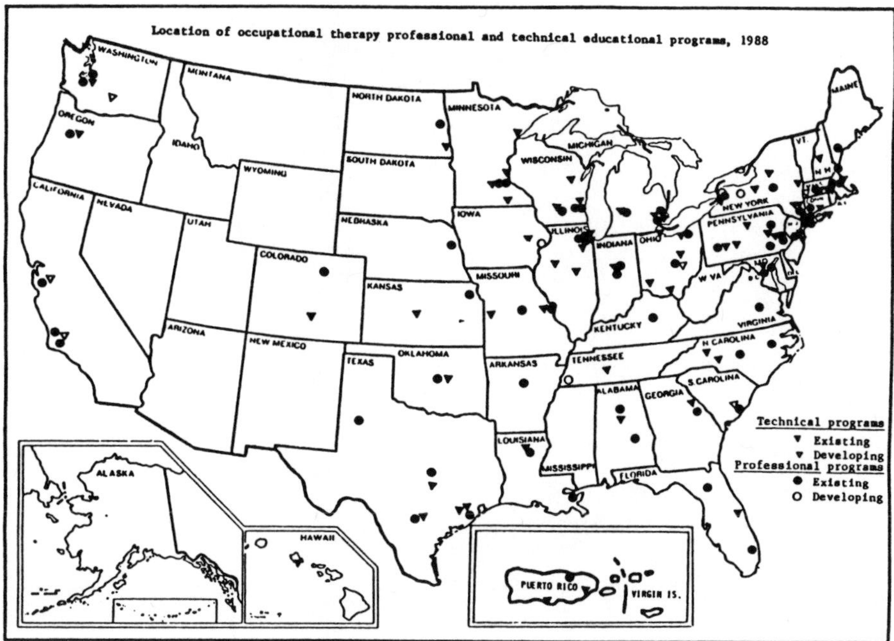

Figure 4-1: Map of the United States showing location of educational programs accredited or approved by the American Occupational Therapy Association or developing toward such status.[13]

Source: 1989 Education Data Survey; AOTA.

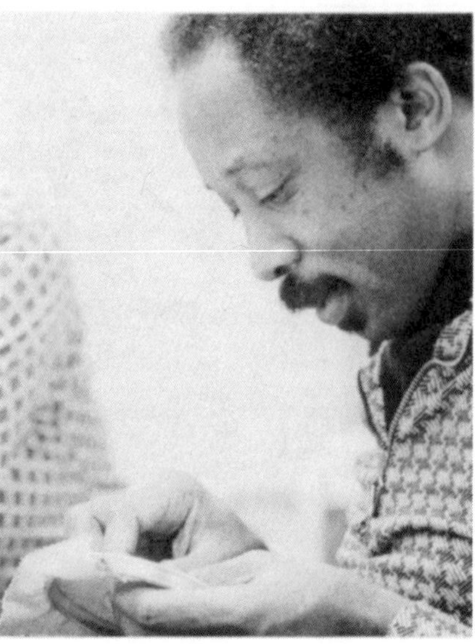

Figure 4-2: In this photo an occupational therapy assistant student learns a needlecraft technique.

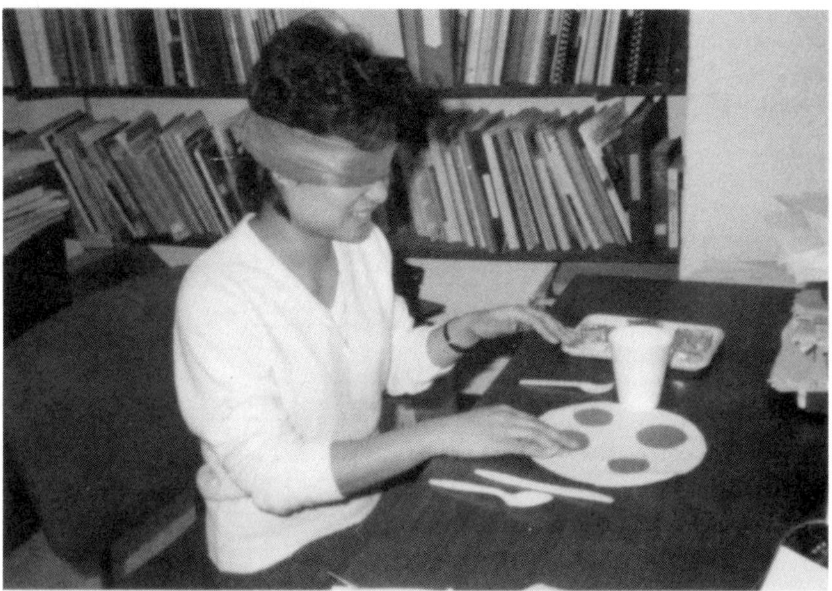

Figure 4-3: The blindfolded occupational therapy assistant student is shown learning to identify a method of placement for the blind.

Years of Education and Training Beyond High School For Careers in Health Occupations

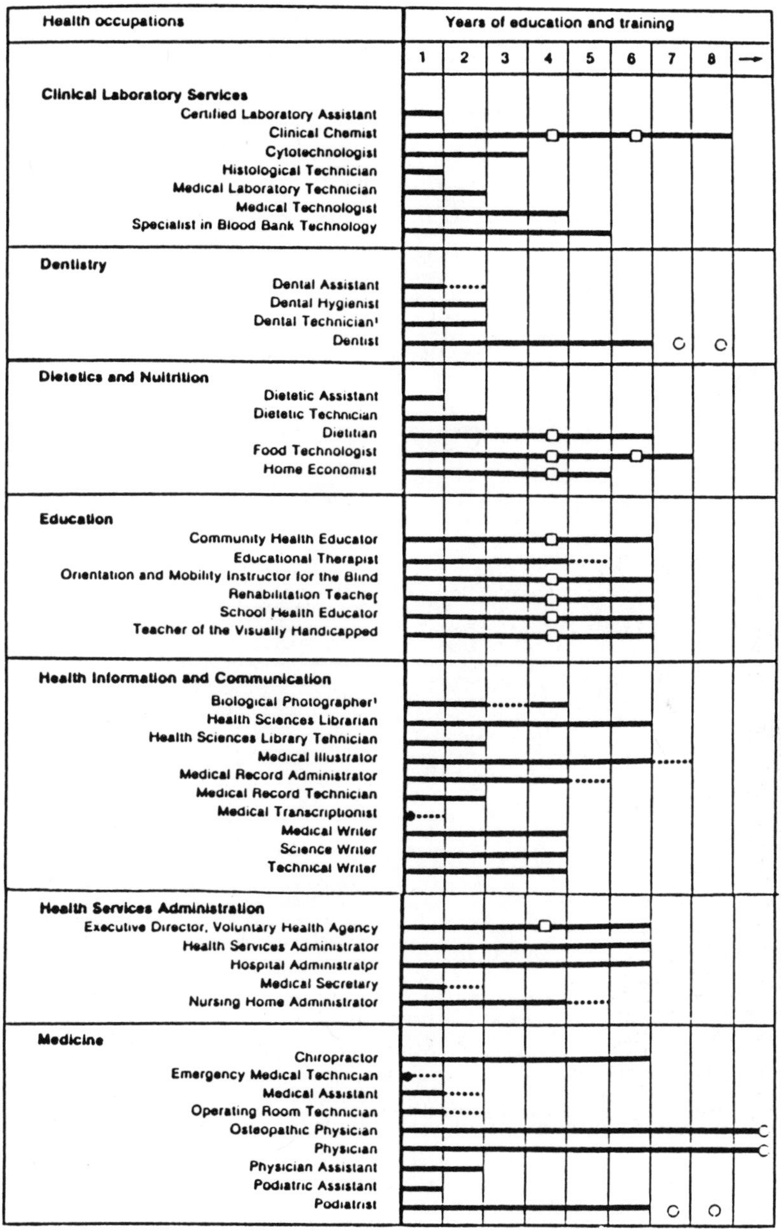

Health occupations	Years of education and training							
	1	2	3	4	5	6	7	8	→
Clinical Laboratory Services									
Certified Laboratory Assistant									
Clinical Chemist									
Cytotechnologist									
Histological Technician									
Medical Laboratory Technician									
Medical Technologist									
Specialist in Blood Bank Technology									
Dentistry									
Dental Assistant									
Dental Hygienist									
Dental Technician[1]									
Dentist									
Dietetics and Nutrition									
Dietetic Assistant									
Dietetic Technician									
Dietitian									
Food Technologist									
Home Economist									
Education									
Community Health Educator									
Educational Therapist									
Orientation and Mobility Instructor for the Blind									
Rehabilitation Teacher									
School Health Educator									
Teacher of the Visually Handicapped									
Health Information and Communication									
Biological Photographer[1]									
Health Sciences Librarian									
Health Sciences Library Tehnician									
Medical Illustrator									
Medical Record Administrator									
Medical Record Technician									
Medical Transcriptionist									
Medical Writer									
Science Writer									
Technical Writer									
Health Services Administration									
Executive Director, Voluntary Health Agency									
Health Services Administrator									
Hospital Administrator									
Medical Secretary									
Nursing Home Administrator									
Medicine									
Chiropractor									
Emergency Medical Technician									
Medical Assistant									
Operating Room Technician									
Osteopathic Physician									
Physician									
Physician Assistant									
Podiatric Assistant									
Podiatrist									

Years of Education and Training Beyond High School For Careers in Health Occupations

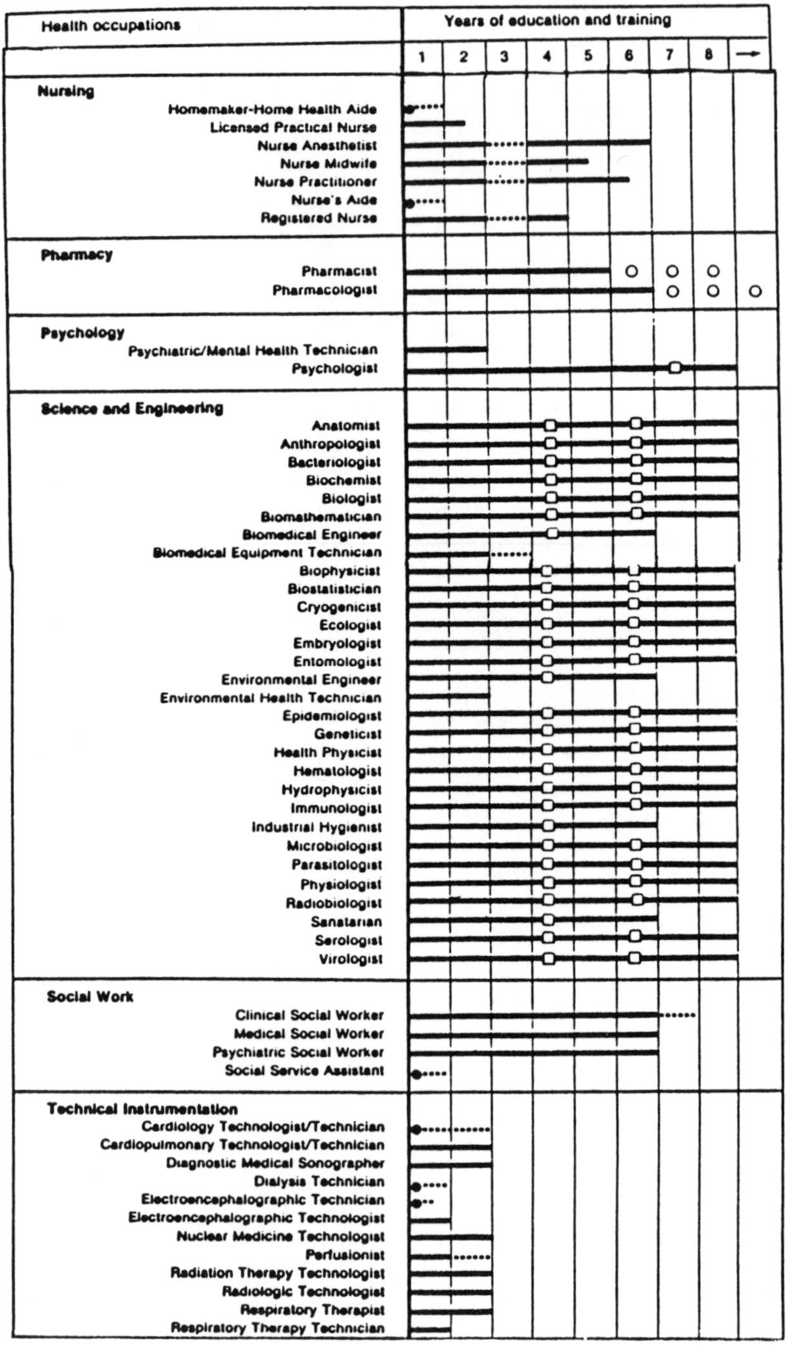

Health occupations	1	2	3	4	5	6	7	8	→
Nursing									
Homemaker-Home Health Aide									
Licensed Practical Nurse									
Nurse Anesthetist									
Nurse Midwife									
Nurse Practitioner									
Nurse's Aide									
Registered Nurse									
Pharmacy									
Pharmacist									
Pharmacologist									
Psychology									
Psychiatric/Mental Health Technician									
Psychologist									
Science and Engineering									
Anatomist									
Anthropologist									
Bacteriologist									
Biochemist									
Biologist									
Biomathematician									
Biomedical Engineer									
Biomedical Equipment Technician									
Biophysicist									
Biostatistician									
Cryogenicist									
Ecologist									
Embryologist									
Entomologist									
Environmental Engineer									
Environmental Health Technician									
Epidemiologist									
Geneticist									
Health Physicist									
Hematologist									
Hydrophysicist									
Immunologist									
Industrial Hygienist									
Microbiologist									
Parasitologist									
Physiologist									
Radiobiologist									
Sanatarian									
Serologist									
Virologist									
Social Work									
Clinical Social Worker									
Medical Social Worker									
Psychiatric Social Worker									
Social Service Assistant									
Technical Instrumentation									
Cardiology Technologist/Technician									
Cardiopulmonary Technologist/Technician									
Diagnostic Medical Sonographer									
Dialysis Technician									
Electroencephalographic Technician									
Electroencephalographic Technologist									
Nuclear Medicine Technologist									
Perfusionist									
Radiation Therapy Technologist									
Radiologic Technologist									
Respiratory Therapist									
Respiratory Therapy Technician									

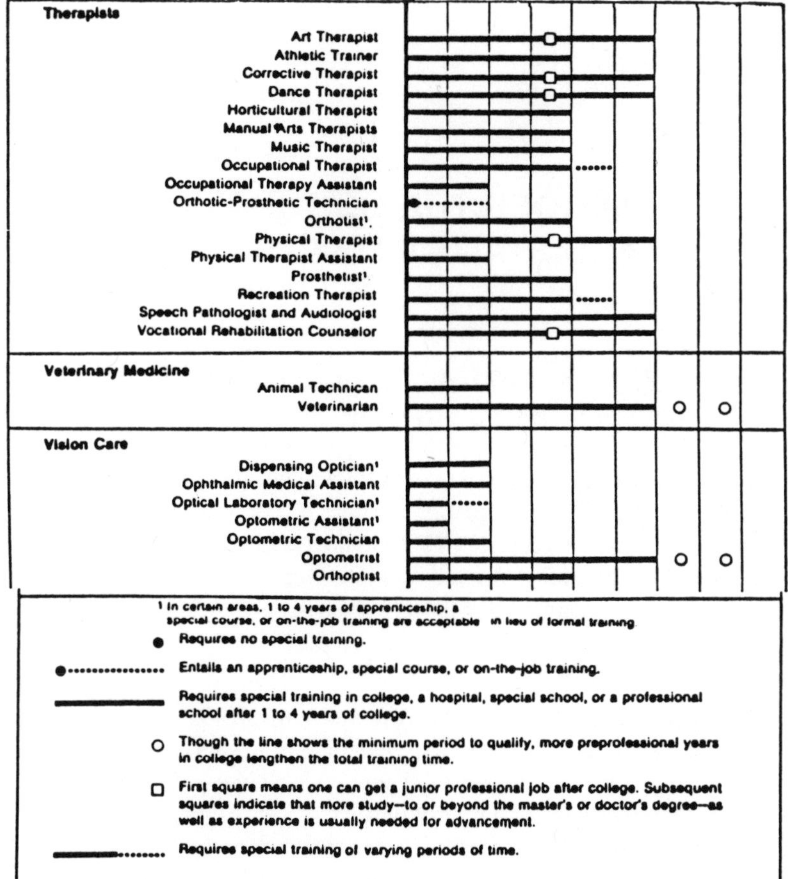

Figure 4-4: *From* Health Careers Guidebook, U.S. Department of Labor, Washington, D.C., U.S. Government Printing Office.[19]

CHAPTER 5

WITH WHOM DOES THE OCCUPATIONAL THERAPY ASSISTANT WORK?

OCCUPATIONAL THERAPY PERSONNEL AND THE HEALTH PROFESSIONALS WITH WHOM THEY WORK

There are two major categories of occupational (OT) therapy personnel certified by the American Occupational Therapy Association. These are the registered occupational therapist (OTR) and the certified occupational therapy assistant (COTA). In addition, many classifications of occupational therapy personnel include an occupational therapy aide.

Occupational Therapist

Training programs for occupational therapists are provided in institutions of higher education and grant either a baccalaureate or master's degree. Students preparing for a bachelor's degree in occupational therapy enter the program either after completion of high school or after completing 2 years of college. Students preparing for a basic master's degree in occupational therapy enter the graduate program after having earned a bachelor's or higher degree in another subject. Both of these routes are considered entry level programs as opposed to graduate training for those already in the field.

In an occupational therapy department a registered occupational therapist might provide services independently or supervise or work with other occupational therapists, occupational therapy assistants or aides. Sometimes a large department headed by an occupational therapist might have several different kinds of personnel. Activities departments or activities therapy departments, for example, could be directed by an occupational therapist or by others and employ activity leaders, recreation therapists, art therapists, music therapists, instructors, dance or movement therapists, craft specialists and horticulture therapists as well as occupational therapists.

The professional level training for the occupational therapist requires a minimum of 6 months of supervised clinical experience to be carried out in at least 2 different settings. Thus the baccalaureate level training generally requires 4-1/2 academic years post high school and the master's degree training

2-1/2 academic years at the graduate level, including both the classroom and clinical components.

Those who are already OTRs may take advanced level occupational therapy specialized education at the master's degree and doctoral degree levels. In 1984 the first Ph.D. in Occupational Therapy was awarded. Many occupational therapists hold master's and doctoral degrees in other fields which enhance their knowledge and practice in specialty areas.

The American Occupational Therapy Association (AOTA) offers a certification examination twice yearly. Students who have graduated from baccalaureate level or master's degree level programs approved by the Association are eligible to sit for the examination. In addition foreign trained occupational therapists who have worked under the supervision of an OTR in this country for one year are also eligible to take the examination. Those who successfully complete the examination are eligible to use the initials OTR (occupational therapist, registered).

In 1989 there were 67 occupational therapy professional programs accredited by the AOTA in conjunction with the American Medical Association (AMA).

The occupational therapist works in a variety of health care, educational and industrial settings as well as in private practice. The primary health problems of patients seen most frequently by OTRs were cerebral vascular accident (stroke), psychosis and cerebral palsy but practice is expanding in new areas. Clients are referred to occupational therapists from a variety of sources. There are occupational therapists listed in classified telephone directories and in directories of practitioners covered under particular forms of health insurance reimbursement policies.

Occupational Therapy Assistant

This category of occupational therapy personnel is described in Chapter 2, and examples are provided throughout the book.

Occupational Therapy Aide

The occupational therapy aide is assigned to the occupational therapy department to primarily carry out support tasks. These might include transporting patients, for example: moving wheelchairs between the occupational therapy department and a patient's floor; preparing or setting up projects or materials such as art supplies; or distributing refreshments during a scheduled activity. In states which have licensure of occupational therapy, aides are not legally permitted to carry out direct occupational therapy services. In states without licensure occupational therapy aides might be found assisting in activities which maintain abilities already achieved by patients or in programs which prevent further deterioration. In the early years occupational therapists were often responsible for diversional therapy. Now occupational therapy aides may distribute projects to keep a patient occupied, but more often this is the responsibility of another department such as recreation.

The occupational therapy aide is generally trained on-the-job perhaps through in-service training. However, there are actual short term training programs for occupational therapy aides as well. In addition there are training programs for rehabilitation aides. Graduates of such programs often take jobs in an occupational therapy department. They might assist a patient in removing or replacing therapeutic appliances such as braces or hand splints, help to adjust wheelchairs or other pieces of equipment or assist in maintaining specialized devices or equipment.

THE HEALTH CARE TEAM

The health care team includes others who work with the occupational therapy assistant. In settings where rehabilitation medicine is the emphasis, the occupational therapy assistant will work with physical therapists and perhaps physical therapist assistants who include in their treatment techniques physical modalities such as ultrasound, heat and cold, electrical stimulation and massage, therapeutic exercise, hydrotherapy (such as whirlpool), ambulation (walking) and mobility training. The physiatrist, the physician who specializes in physical medicine and rehabilitation, generally refers patients to both physical and occupational therapy. The physiatrist completes a 3 year residency training period after medical school, while the physical therapist is trained at the baccalaureate degree or master's degree level and the physical therapist assistant generally at the associate degree or community college level.

In mental health settings the physician responsible is the psychiatrist who completes a residency in psychiatry or community mental health following four years of medical school which in turn follows four years of college. The psychiatrist may use psychotherapy, as might the psychiatric social worker or the psychologist, but is the only member of the treatment team who can prescribe medications or use electro shock therapy. The social worker earns a Master of Social Work degree and is generally the team member who meets with the family or significant other to plan for the patient's discharge or to deal with home arrangements during the treatment period. The clinical psychologist generally holds a Ph.D. or Doctor of Psychology degree and may be involved in testing to determine particular areas in which the patient has deficits.

Both the social worker and psychologist are found in all areas of occupational therapy practice. This is also true of nursing staff. The registered nurse may be trained at the associate degree or baccalaureate degree level and may take on special roles in varying areas of practice. The rehabilitation nurse may focus on self care including, for example, training a spinal cord injured patient to deal with toileting needs. The psychiatric nurse may lead group sessions.

The occupational therapy assistant also works with the vocational rehabilitation counselor in a variety of settings. With training generally at the master's degree level the vocational rehabilitation counselor may be involved in placing the client in actual employment, arranging for funding support during a training program geared to employment, or perhaps directing a vocational testing unit of a workshop.

The speech therapist generally holds a master's degree and may work closely with occupational therapy personnel on feeding programs where swallowing is important, in stroke rehabilitation where speech deficits often accompany the disability and in promoting communication in a variety of conditions.

Occupational therapy assistants work with other physicians in specialty areas of practice. These include particularly the orthopedist, the cardiologist, the pediatrician and the geriatrician. Their key areas of practice related to OT respectively are: fractures and hand rehabilitation, heart disease with energy conservation and activity tolerance, developmental disorders and birth defects or childhood accidents, and various concerns related to aging.

Some members of the health care team work directly in occupational therapy departments or under the direction on occupational therapy personnel.

Activity therapy staff often work under the direction of an occupational therapist who may head the activity therapy department. Activity therapy departments, particularly in psychiatric centers, may include within them occupational therapists, music therapists, art therapists, dance therapists and other activity therapists. These individuals are usually credentialed by their national associations after completing baccalaureate or master's degree programs in their specialty areas.

Activities departments in settings such as nursing homes may be directed by occupational therapy assistants. The director is generally called "Activities Program Director" whether the person is an occupational therapy assistant or from another background such as activity leadership, recreation or one of the creative arts therapies. The director is responsible for supervising activity leaders who may be trained in one of the specialty areas mentioned above or who may have special skills, such as arts and crafts, or group leadership. Volunteers are also generally an important part of an activities program and may be particularly skilled in a needed area or just have the interest in assisting with scheduled activities.

COMPARISON BETWEEN OTR AND COTA

Education and Certification

The initials OTR stand for Occupational Therapist, Registered. These initials are designated by the AOTA for use by an individual who has met eligibility requirements including completion of an accredited curriculum in occupational therapy. Professional occupational therapy programs are accredited jointly by the AOTA and the American Medical Association. These programs might be either at the bachelor's degree (4 years) or master's degree (graduate school) level. Following completion of the program, the graduate may sit for the national certification examination established by the AOTA. Upon successful completion including a minimum of 6 months fieldwork the individual is eligible for certification and use of the initials OTR.

COTA refers to Certified Occupational Therapy Assistant. These initials are designated by the AOTA and may only be used by individuals who meet the organization's requirements. These requirements include successful completion of an approved occupational therapy assistant curriculum with a minimum of 2 months fieldwork. Such programs are approved by the AOTA as meeting its standards for Essentials of an Occupational Therapy Assistant Training Program. These programs vary in length. The AOTA passed a resolution encouraging OTA programs to be at the associate degree level, and the new Essentials require that OTA education be in post secondary educational institutions. Certificate programs are nine months to one year in length. After completion of the program the graduate is eligible for the national certification examination. Upon passing the examination the individual is eligible for certification by the AOTA and subsequent use of the initials COTA. Table 5-1 provides a general comparison.

Practice

The above paragraphs describe the differences in education and eligibility for using the initials COTA and OTR. There are differences in practice as well. The American Occupational Therapy Association has conducted several studies and released information on role differentiation between the two levels in Occupational Therapy. The AOTA role delineation study emphasizes that the entry level COTA (during the first year of practice) is under the supervision of the OTR and assists in many areas which the OTR actually plans, analyzes, and interprets. The major areas of the role delineation document are referral, occupational therapy treatment, discontinuation, service management, continued education, and public relations. Both the COTA and the OTR participate in all of these areas. In some settings the COTA functions independently on a day to day basis with the OTR coming in periodically as a consultant. In many cases there is no OTA in the setting, and, where there are both an OTR and COTA, differences may depend on the level of training and experience of the COTA. The 1981 Role Delineation[17] document is included in the Appendix. Table 4-2 provides an overview.

Since there are continuing questions regarding practice issues in occupational therapy, the AOTA Division of Practice has established a column in "Occupational Therapy News" entitled "I'm Glad You Asked." Recent responses about the occupational therapy assistant in relation to the OTR have included: (1) "The AOTA does not mandate that a *referral* from a physician be obtained to initiate occupational therapy services. The statement on Occupational Therapy Referral states: 'The registered occupational therapist (OTR) and the certified occupational therapy assistant (COTA) respond to a request for services whatsoever its source. The OTR enters a case at his or her own professional discretion on his or her own cognizance. The COTA enters as authorized by the supervising OTR.'...However, a referral may be required by the policies of your facility, voluntary accrediting agencies, federal law, third party reimbursers, or OT State licensure laws." (2) "COTAs are recognized by AOTA...as qualified to write notes in patients' charts. The current AOTA guidelines do not require that COTA notes be countersigned...but it is a recognized method of documenting supervision." (3) "There are no standards that dictate the minimum amount of time necessary to supervise a COTA. The AOTA document 'Guide for Supervision of OT Personnel' recommends that an entry level COTA receive close supervision and that a more experienced COTA be provided general supervision...Medicare regulations define general supervision as 'initial direction and periodic inspection of the actual activity; however, the supervisor need not always be physically present or on the premises when the assistant is performing services'...State licensure acts include very general supervision guidelines regarding COTA's."

Figure 5-1 shows occupational therapy personnel working together.

IN THE WORDS OF AN OCCUPATIONAL THERAPY ASSISTANT

Rehab, Inc. is an agency equipped to service rehabilitation centers, nursing homes, public health agencies, and private homes. Its multidisciplinary team provides: social work, rehabilitation nursing, speech therapy, physical therapy, and occupational therapy.

We are 3 OTRs and 2 COTAs. My role is to assist the OTR in attaining maximum restoration of patients abilities. Some of my functions are: administer patients' treatment programs; construct splints; participate in patient evaluation meetings; order equipment and supplies and maintain department inventory; write progress notes, summaries, and discharge summaries.

A very important factor, which makes my job much more effective, is that the nursing staff is interested in the patient's progress in the rehabilitation program and is very cooperative with rehabilitation staff.

I think this is essential for an effective rehabilitation program and I am pleased to work with a professional team.

Marilena Andrade, COTA
Rehab, Inc.
Washington, D.C.

IN THE WORDS OF OCCUPATIONAL THERAPY ASSISTANTS

As COTAs, we have worked in the Beaverton, Oregon School District through a contract with Saint Vincent Hospital and Medical Center for two-and-a-half years. We are part of the motor development team that also includes adaptive physical education specialists, occupational therapists, registered physical therapists, and licensed physical therapist assistants (LPTA). This team serves 44 schools and approximately 500 students ranging from 3 to 21 years of age.

The OTR and COTA work together and balance and coordinate their services by using each person's strength and specific educational backgrounds. We have comparable caseloads of students with physical disabilities, developmental disabilities, mental retardation, learning disabilities, emotional disturbances, language disorders, sensory impairments, and other health impairments. The COTA works in various settings such as self-contained classrooms, resource rooms, and regular and special programs.

Then what makes an OTR an OTR and a COTA a COTA? Both the COTA and OTR provide direct treatment, consultation, screening, testing, information gathering, statistical data, and inservices. They are both members of the motor team and serve as a role model for both OT and OTA students. The OTR role responsibilities include developing policies and procedures for service, determining student eligibility for service, communicating to physicians, report writing, equipment design, determining needs for changes in student programs, and supervising assistants. The COTA's specific responsibilities are to keep inventory, fabricate equipment, order supplies, record services, and provide guides for recreational and community resources. Training students in activities of daily living (such as prevocation, feeding, and dressing skills), incorporating motor function (gross and fine), sensori-perceptual motor integration, and crafts in activity performance are forms of treatment given by the COTA.

In the Beaverton School District COTAs are usually involved from the beginning to the end of the student's treatment process. After the motor team receives a referral for a student, the COTA along with the LPTA does a pre-evaluation (i.e., information gathering, screening, and testing). Results are passed onto the OTR and the rest of the team prior to the formal evaluation. This process addresses areas of concern, decreases formal evaluation time, and provides the COTA with hands on experience in the evaluation. An IEP (individual education plan) meeting is then held. The COTA attends this meeting when involved in providing student services. Then the student is seen in the various classroom settings. Different forms of treatment are used depending on the students' individual needs (i.e., group treatment with other disciplines, individual one-to-one therapy, and/or parallel treatment with the OTR). The COTA and the OTR then review the student's needs, discuss student's progress to determine the level of service, formulate new goals, and establish revised treatment plans when necessary.

Our unique role as COTAs provides opportunities to contribute and share our skills and knowledge as paraprofessionals. We have specific and special skills to contribute and are necessary and vital members of the treatment team.*

Niki Phillipe, COTA
Micki Walker, COTA[22]
Beaverton, Oregon School District

SUGGESTIONS

1. Talk with people working in different areas of the health field.
2. Form your own impressions about key aspects and differences in their occupations.
3. Speak to both an occupational therapist and occupational therapy assistant or student about their impressions of their own roles and those of others within occupational therapy.
4. Write to the American Occupational Therapy Association for information about both the occupational therapist and the occupational therapy assistant.

READING OBJECTIVES

1. Explain ways in which the occupational therapy assistant differs from the occupational therapist in education, practice and certification.

*The full article, entitled "COTA and OTR Treatment Team in Schools" appeared in Occupational Therapy News, October 1984.

2. Name other members of the health care team with whom the occupational therapy assistant works and an example of a function of each.
3. Identify a trend in occupational therapy manpower.
4. Give examples of other personnel who might work in an occupational therapy department.

REFERENCES

[17]American Occupational Therapy Association: Entry-Level OTR and COTA Role Delineation, 1981.

[18]American Occupational Therapy Association: Essentials for an Educational Program for OTA, 1983.

[19]Health Careers Guidebook, U.S. Dept. of Labor, 1978.

[20]American Occupational Therapy Association: Fieldwork Evaluation Form for Occupational Therapy Assistants, 1983.

[21]Davis L: Update—ROTE Project. Gerontology Special Interest Newsletter 7:3, 1984.

[22]Phillipe N, Walker M: COTA and OTR Treatment Team in Schools. Occupational Therapy News. October, 1984.

TABLE 5-1
A GENERAL COMPARISON BETWEEN THE OTR AND COTA IN EDUCATION AND CERTIFICATION

OTR	*COTA*
EDUCATION	
Senior College or graduate school	Postsecondary education institution, generally community or junior college
Baccalaureate degree (BS/BA) or basic Master's degree	Certificate or Associate degree (AS/AAS/AA)
Minimum of 4 academic years post high school	Nine months to 2 years after high school
Can enter with high school diploma or equivalency or previous college or degree	Can enter with high school diploma or equivalency or previous college or degree
Program accredited by AOTA with American Medical Association	Program approved by (AOTA) American Occupational Therapy Association
Six months advanced level supervised fieldwork (minimum)	Two months advanced level supervised fieldwork (minimum)
Content areas in accordance with AOTA Essentials of an Education Program for the Occupational Therapist	Content areas in accordance with AOTA Essentials of an Education Program for the Occupational Therapy Assistant
CERTIFICATION CRITERIA	
Graduation from an accredited educational program	Graduation from an approved educational program
Successfully completing 6 months of fieldwork	Successfully completing 2 months of fieldwork
Successfully completing the national certification examination for OTR offered twice a year	Successfully completing the national certification examination for COTA offered twice a year

TABLE 5-2
A COMPARISON IN ROLES AND FUNCTIONS OF OCCUPATIONAL THERAPIST AND OCCUPATIONAL THERAPY ASSISTANT DURING FIRST YEAR OF PRACTICE*

	Therapist	*Assistant*
Referral	Responds	Responds and relays to OTR
	Initiates	Initiates for daily living skills
	Supervises documentation	Enters case as authorized by OTR
	Delegates to COTA	
Occupational Therapy Assessment	SCREENING	
	Collect data	Collect data
	Analyze data	Organize data
	Formulate recommendations	
	Document and report	
	EVALUATION	
	Select areas to evaluate	
	Plan methodology	
	Explain plan	
	Interview	Assist by interviewing with structured format
	Observe	Assist by observing during activity
	Administer assessments	Administer structured tests
	Analyze and synthesize data	
	Document interpretation	Summarize own data to supervisor
	Report	Report as determined by OTR
	Develop recommendations	Make recommendations to OTR
Program Planning	Develop goals	Assist OTR with development of goals
	Refer client	
	Select OT techniques and media	Assist OTR in selecting techniques and media
	Analyze components	Analyze activities in selected areas
	Adapt techniques and media	Adapt techniques and media under supervision
	Discuss OT goals and methods	Discuss OT goals and methods
	Document and report	Document and report as directed by OTR
	Coordinate the program	
	Determine point of termination	
Occupational Therapy Treatment	Engage client in purposeful activity to achieve goals[2]	Under direction of OTR, engage client in purposeful activity to achieve goals[2]
	Orient and instruct others	Orient and instruct others
	Observe precautions	Observe precautions
	Prepare and instruct home program	Assist in instruction of home program developed by OTR
	Monitor client's program[2]	Monitor client's program[2]

Program Discontinuation	Formulate discharge and follow-up plan	Discuss need for discontinuation with OTR
	Recommend termination of OT services	
	Prepare home program	Assist OTR in preparing home program
	Recommend adaptations	Assist OTR in recommending adaptations
	Refer client and/or family	
	Recommend community resources	Assist OTR in identifying community resources
	Summarize and document	Assist in summarizing and documenting
	Terminate program	
Service Management	Maintain service[2]	Maintain service[2]
	Recruit, select, orient, train, supervise and evaluate personnel	Assist with other personnel
	Plan, direct, coordinate and evaluate service programs	Assist OTR with evaluation of service program
	Determine service and personnel needs	
	Assure collaboration and communication	
	Develop and implement quality review	Participate in quality review program
	Participate in accrediting reviews	Participate in accrediting reviews
	Supervise students	Supervise students as assigned by OTR
	Develop justification for OT services	
Continued Education	Participate in continuing education	Participate in continuing education
	Participate in inservice programs	Participate in inservice programs
	Plan and provide inservice education	Assist OTR in planning and providing inservice education
Public Relations	Identify need for and explain OT	Explain occupational therapy
	Serve as a representative of OT	Serve as a representative of OT

*Based on Entry-Level Role Delineation for OTRs and COTAs, American Occupational Therapy Association, March 1981.

[2]See specific areas identified in Role Delineation document in Appendix.

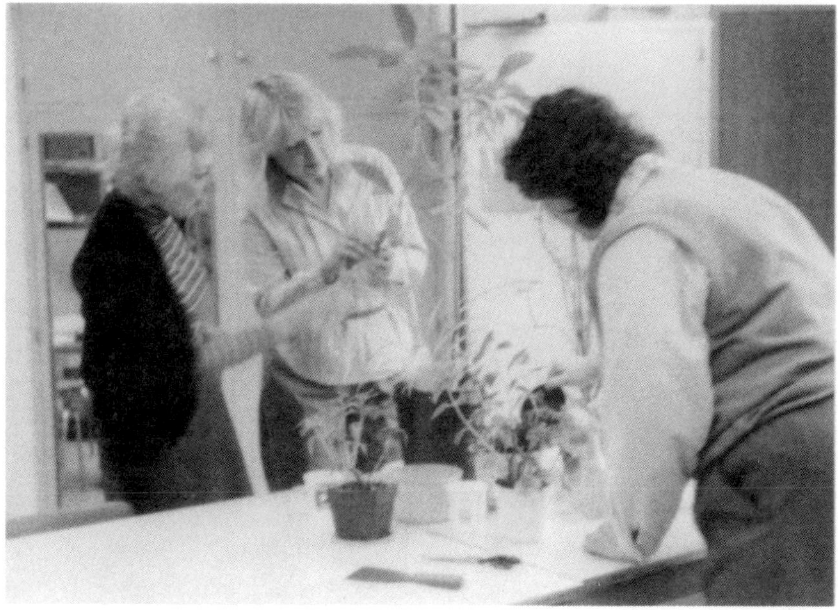

Figure 5-1: Collaboration among occupational therapy staff is the key to success. Here an OTR who is a former COTA, a COTA and an OTA student (left to right) prepare for a gardening group.

PART II

OCCUPATIONAL THERAPY ASSISTANTS IN PRACTICE

CHAPTER 6

THE OCCUPATIONAL THERAPY ASSISTANT WORKS WITH THE AGED

THE OCCUPATIONAL THERAPY ASSISTANT AND THE AGED

Who are the Aged?

The aged are most often defined as those over the age of 65. Individuals are sometimes grouped into this category based on health, appearance, behavior, personality, or dependence. Retirement communities often limit entrance to those over 55, and many medical facilities for the aged actually house primarily those over 75. Individuals age differently. The field of geriatrics refers to the medical aspects of the aged. Gerontology refers to the all encompassing study of the aged.

Of the 20 million people in the United States who are age 65 or older (more than 11% of the population) only 5% are institutionalized. The aged often have problems in several areas, rather than just one, and they are more likely to have illnesses with long-term effects.

Where is Occupational Therapy for the Aged Provided?

Nursing homes employ the greatest number of occupational therapy assistants. The term nursing home is used for a variety of in-patient or residential facilities. The most intensive medical care for the elderly is provided by acute or general hospitals. The Skilled Nursing Facility (SNF) emphasizes professional nursing care and can admit patients for rehabilitation services. Skilled Nursing Facilities are generally called nursing homes. The Health Related Facility (HRF) serves those who need less specialized care. It is often called a Health Care Center. Board and Care Homes or Homes for the Aged provide a place to live, meals, cleaning and simple personal assistance. Activities Programs are also sometimes available in such institutions. The aged are also found in day care programs and home health programs where services might range from providing specialized treatment to support services to help the person maintain abilities and thereby continue to live in the community.

How Will I Train to be an Occupational Therapy Assistant with the Aged?

Particularly in later years, physical, psychological and social aspects of the elderly patient's life are all effected when there is a change in one area. For example: if an elderly person breaks a leg, confinement to a room might lead to feeling lonely and depressed. Therefore, most of what is learned in an occupational therapy assistant training program is important when treating an aged person. OTAs should know of the changes which occur in the systems of the body as well as psychological and social changes that take place as a person gets older. Some of this knowledge comes from courses in normal developmental processes, anatomy and physiology.

Training in therapeutic activities and skills is particularly important when working with the aged. A variety of general crafts are used in activities programs for this group. Woodworking is easily adapted to improve physical limitations. Group dynamic skills enable the occupational therapy assistant to lead groups to achieve such goals as socialization. "Activities of Daily Living" knowledge is used in every geriatric setting whether for specific instructions in self care approaches or for encouragement of personal hygiene and grooming for self esteem. This might include adapting tasks, modifying equipment or positioning the aged individual as well as demonstrating specific techniques related to dressing, feeding or grooming.

In Practice

Recognizing this growing area of practice as important for the future, the American Occupational Therapy Association set up Project ROTE (the Role of Occupational Therapy with the Elderly).[21] The first phase of the project showed that there appears to be considerable overlap in role functions of OTRs, COTAs, and related practitioners in dealing with the aged.

Thus both OTRs and COTAs were eligible for the faculty to lead regional ROTE workshops for OTRs and COTAs during 1986 and Occupational Therapy Assistant educational program faculty were trained in 1987. In 1983 the American Occupational Therapy Association adopted a position paper and guidelines covering occupational therapy and activity programs in long term care—the major areas of function for the occupational therapy assistant in geriatrics or aging. It emphasized that OT activities differ in "(a) the purpose for which the activity is used, (b) the process of selecting activity, (c) the role of interests in the selection process, and (d) the scope of services." It clarified that in occupational therapy the OTR maintains supervisory responsibility for all tasks delegated to the COTA while the COTA may function independently in conducting activities programs. Figure 6-1 depicts a specific occupational therapy approach. Following are actual examples of occupational therapy assistants and occupational therapy assistant students in practice with the aged.

EXAMPLES OF OCCUPATIONAL THERAPY ASSISTANTS WORKING WITH THE AGED

Skilled Nursing Facility

Gladys, a recent graduate of an associate degree program, works in a well structured occupational therapy rehabilitation department in a small nursing home. She is one of three occupational therapy staff members. One of her patients is a man who never married and was always dependent on his younger sister. He had served as a messenger for people in the community. At the age of 72 he suffered a stroke (cerebral vascular accident), and his sister felt that she could no longer care for him. He was admitted to the nursing home with hemiplegia (half sided paralysis), severely impaired judgement, and periods of confusion and forgetfulness. He wore eye glasses and his hearing was poor. He was evaluated by the occupational therapist in the following areas with results as noted:

Range of Motion—limitations in right shoulder and in elbow extension

Muscle Strength—right arm and hand weakness

Sensation—decreased sensation on right side

Functional Use—right hand used for writing, minor tasks and to propel wheelchair; left side is normal

Activities of Daily Living—dependent, refuses to try shaving and dressing

Transfer Abilities—requires minimal assistance to stand and transfer from wheelchair to chair.

The following goals were established:

1. Improve ability to transfer from wheelchair to chair
2. Improve ability to perform activities of daily living including shaving and dressing
3. Increase muscle strength in the arms and hands
4. Improve wheelchair management
5. Increase attention span
6. Decrease perceptual problems during performance of tasks

Gladys scheduled the patient twice each week for occupational therapy to meet the therapeutic goals. She demonstrated to the patient how to stand from his wheelchair using proper body mechanics and safety techniques and then to transfer to a straight chair. Stating the steps verbally, she instructed the patient in dressing and grooming techniques which took into account his limited strength and range of motion on his right side. He was, for example, shown how to position his shirt on his lap so that his right hand could be slid easily into the sleeve opening. He practiced the steps under the direction of the occupational therapy assistant. The patient also began a woodworking project to increase strength, improve attention span and reduce perceptual problems.

Initially the patient resisted treatment but as Gladys developed a positive relationship with him, he cooperated and improved in all areas.

Psychiatric Center

Marcella enjoys being a COTA in the geriatric unit of a large state psychiatric center since she is one of ten staff members in the occupational therapy department. She sees herself as being able to meet the department's goals of enhancing total social development, work skills and independent functioning of patients toward future community living. She finds it an advantage to be an occupational therapy assistant in this setting where she is given full responsibility for a ward with regard to planning the activity program and can supervise beginning OTA students. Marcella first worked as an aide in this setting and found out first hand that encouragement is a valuable tool for increasing motivation. Her OT supervisors encouraged her to return to school and were able to adjust her work schedule so that she could continue to earn while pursuing her OTA career through part-time schooling.

An example of one of Marcella's patients is a 70 year old widow. To increase her self esteem and level of independence the patient was assigned limited tasks in the workshop. By completing the specific task in the assigned time she achieved a feeling of accomplishment. For example, she would complete two crocheted potholders and hang them on a wall for all to admire giving her self-gratification, or she would complete a ceramic piece which increased her self autonomy.

It is also important that the patient be given tasks which give her the feeling that she is a responsible individual, such as wiping off the tables after each workshop session. Marcella's patient had always needed reassurance. To increase and develop her independent function, she was asked to assist in group sessions. The COTA assigned the patient a role involving preparation for this group activity which helped the patient develop trust in others. She was also given finger painting as therapeutic activity to help her to express her feelings through colors. Communication was also enhanced through this activity, particularly during discussion following the finger painting experience.

The patient attended occupational therapy 1/2 hour each morning four days each week. At each session she was given a specific task such as stuffing a pillow and was also given a specific responsibility to complete on a daily basis after workshop, for example clearing the tables.

Independent Living Center

Helen is a COTA who works in an Independent Living Center for older individuals who are blind or have visual impairment. One of her typical patients was a man with severe visual impairment as a result of glaucoma, right sided weakness from a previous stroke, and diabetes. To improve his independence in self care and activities of daily living, Helen initiated both a group and individual occupational therapy program.

In the area of eating the patient was asked to explore the table setting (identifying through touch, taste, smell and hearing, the salt, pepper, knife, and other table items) and locate the food and identify it using a fork and senses. The patient learned to use a rocker knife (with rounded sharp edge) for cutting meat with only one hand. The patient was also introduced to the metal plate guard and its application and effectiveness in loading and keeping food on the plate. In a food group for the blind, the patient learned such activities as buttering bread with softened butter and pouring hot and cold liquids. To enable the patient to pour hot and cold liquids Helen broke down the activity into specific steps. The patient learned to pour efficiently starting with cold water and plastic mugs. First the mug to be filled was held stationary on a special material for the purpose or on a wet paper towel. The patient ran the index finger of his left hand down the inner surface of the glass to the level of the liquid, alternating his left hand first as the indicator and then as the pouring hand. To compensate for loss of sensation, the patient touched his index finger to his lips and face to determine whether it was wet.

For food preparation the COTA had the patient learn to identify foods by touch, smell and taste; by wrapping rubber bands around can products; by raised labels; and by organizing foods by categories. In a group, the patient learned the use and care of various kitchen aids designed for the visually impaired, for example, a vegetable chopper, an adapted cutting board and a pocket hand-held magnifier for reading recipes and directions.

On a one-to-one basis with the therapist, the patient learned to use the equipment adapted for his needs (such as built-up handles for utensils, a rocker knife and a long-handle reacher) for efficient food preparation using his left hand. The patient learned cooking safety skills including use of a wooden spoon, centering a pot, detecting heat, and regulation of burners and oven.

After mastering eating and food preparation the patient's program focused on grooming, bathing and washing. The patient was trained by the OTA to identify objects by touching them to face or lips, by odor, and by identifying bands on them. Equipment such as a built-up long handled brush, toothbrush, one-handed buttoner and zipper pull, stocking aid, long handled sponge, hand-held shower nozzle, and toe scrubber were explored in individual sessions with the OTA. The patient also participated in a grooming group, gaining support from others. The patient learned the use of various visual aids available, such as hand-held magnifier with light, as well as application of techniques including good lighting, scanning techniques and visual recall while participating in a group for the visually impaired.

In the area of dressing and clothing maintenance, the COTA trained the patient to coordinate his personal wardrobe by employing an identification system and by hanging all his clothes and polishing his shoes with clear wax. The next step for the patient was to learn to handle money by identifying coins through size and thickness and grouping the same coins in separate compartments of an accordian purse. He learned to discriminate different denominations of paper money by folding techniques. The patient relearned to tell time using a pocket magnifier held at a specified distance directly over the face of a self-winding watch, how to set a large faced alarm clock step by step using a hand-held magnifier, and to orient himself to the time of day by being alert to sounds such as a siren, radio news or recognized T.V. programs. Practice and discussion of new skills took place in groups led by the COTA.

Health Related Facility

Mifa began her career in occupational therapy at an age when most people are planning retirement. Her children were grown and married and she began doing volunteer work in a hospital. She was encouraged by an OTR at her hospital to go to OTA school. Since she already had a master's degree in economics she chose a certificate program. Mifa has a longtime interest in geriatrics and had also taken a course in dance therapy and so began her OT career working part time at a small nursing home. Her job function evolved from working twelve hours per week doing movement therapy and rehabilitation treatment to being the full time director of activities with an OTR serving as consultant two days per week.

Mifa described the basic issues in running activity programs as the need to reach all patients, at all levels; work within a limited budget; and the need to gain cooperation from other departments. She created and directs a dynamic program which, besides arts and crafts and social games, includes movement classes, lectures, newspaper groups, a residents' council and an adopt-a-school program with other nursing homes and organizations in the area. Mifa has coordinated and trained a staff of volunteers to design and lead programs. She has actively sought out actors, dancers and speakers (who work through special funding or volunteer their time) and utilized students in health related fields or college work study programs to enable the activities program to be varied and meaningful to the patients. A great deal of her time is spent on administrative work—coordinating her staff and doing the paperwork involved in dealing with institutions and government agencies; however, Mifa still makes time to work with patients, to contact each one personally, and to encourage them to get involved in the program.

Since more of the well elderly now choose to stay in the community as long as possible, Mifa has had to adjust her activities program accordingly to meet the needs of more seriously physically and emotionally disabled persons. Mifa is committed to her position and continues her education in geriatrics through regular workshops and extensive reading.

Community Outreach Program

Juan services primarily Alzheimer's Disease clients and their families but is also responsible for educating the community to the problems encountered when this disease strikes and to the types of programs available for its victims. Although the position could have been filled by someone with another background, Juan was selected because of his occupational therapy assistant training as well as his interest in the population.

Juan has concentrated his efforts on meeting the specific functional needs of the client or the family. If memory is a concern, for example, he will train both the client and family to use lists and post them prominently, to have large clocks at eye height and to set alarms, and to reduce the amount of instructions given at one time while increasing the repetition. He will also introduce memory games such as Concentration.

Chronic Disease Hospital

Felicity works as a COTA with a variety of patients with long-term conditions. A number of her aged patients suffer from Parkinson's Disease. She has learned to recognize the shuffling gait and lack of facial expression symptomatic of the disease due to muscle impairment. Despite appearances, the Parkinson's Disease patient is quite capable of understanding and handling intellectual activities, as Felicity has learned. She has also learned that the tremor that the Parkinson's Disease patient has when at rest will not be present when actually engaging in an activity. The therapeutic goals for these patients are primarily directed toward maintaining function and preventing deterioration while promoting a positive outlook. Activities include self care and involvement of the hands and mind.

Rehabilitation Center

Marylou is an occupational therapy assistant in a rehabilitation center. She works individually with assigned patients. One typical client was an older man who was active in the field of law until the stroke (cerebral vascular accident) which paralyzed his left side and made speech difficult. The patient was very distressed by these new limitations and was often found in tears. He had also experienced a loss of memory and found concentration difficult. Other patients could not understand his speech which made socializing difficult and he had shoulder pains when walking with his cane and needed help in dressing and eating.

In the course of his treatment Marylou introduced the patient to increasingly more difficult activities which he could still handle. Thus, occupational therapy helped him realize that his situation was not hopeless, that he could cope with the new limitations imposed by half sided paralysis and improve on them, and work towards making full use of the mobility and capability that he still commands.

General Hospital

Joan is a COTA who works in a large medical center. One of her patients was an 83 year old male who was recuperating from a broken hip. Like many aged individuals, he had multiple problems. He was assigned to the OT program five times each week. The immediate goals for the patient were his safety needs and adjustment to his new environment. He was first trained by Joan to get out of his wheelchair without falling and to shift to a regular chair. To do this Joan made him aware of first locking his wheelchair to avoid any accidents. He was also instructed to position his feet correctly under him so he would have enough room to pivot his body while transferring. Since he had a hearing loss, Joan had to speak slowly and face him directly. After meeting the immediate goal, Joan trained him to put on his trousers and to remove his shoes and socks in spite of the limited movement of his hip. To accomplish this Joan instructed him in many of the specialized techniques she had learned during her training, such as having him lie on the bed to remove his slacks. Joan felt great satisfaction when his progress was demonstrated to his family, she saw that the occupational therapy she was providing would enable him to return to them quickly.

Home Care

Amy is the only COTA with a group of occupational and physical therapists who established a home health practice. Her primary case load consists of patients living in the community who have been referred by Visiting Nurse Service, by home health agencies or by private doctors. Occasionally Amy makes a home visit with or for a hospitalized patient who is expected to be discharged back to the community. This might involve checking out the width of doorways or the height of cabinets to assess whether the patient will be able to manage a wheelchair in a particular environment.

Amy deals with both the physical and psychological needs of her clients in the home. She helps them develop leisure activities to productively occupy their many hours alone and trains them in self care activities within their limitations. She also provides for special devices where indicated and carries out therapeutic exercise programs for increasing strength or range of motion within the treatment plan written by the OTR.

Amy must be sensitive to the particular environment of the home including the physical facilities and family members. She uses the trunk of her car as a mobile office. It contains a file cabinet with resource materials, boxes of craft materials, equipment that is small enough to be easily transported, assistive devices for self care, and small items for therapeutic exercise and perception training.

Since she is usually on her own, Amy must be sure she has brought all the necessary items with her, has checked with the OTR in advance regarding any questions, and observes all safety precautions. She likes the feeling of independence she has in home care and the variety of working in a different location each day. Some patients are seen only once for a special need while others are seen one to three times each week.

Senior Center Day Program

Deborah works in a government funded "Service Program for the Aged." It is a day program for older individuals living in the community who are exhibiting signs of confusion, depression, and memory loss. During the morning the program provides therapeutic groups to meet the special needs of these clients including introduction of reality orientation (consistent repetitions focus on the fundamentals of who, what, where, and when) and remotivation groups (in-depth discussion around one topic). In the afternoon it offers programming similar to senior centers including games, recreation, general crafts, and discussion groups. Sensory training is provided as well.

IN THE WORDS OF OCCUPATIONAL THERAPY ASSISTANTS

As COTAs in a long-term care facility, we are proud of our roles, professional image, and the quality of our supportive therapy and activity programs. In developing a variety of programs, our goals are to provide quality treatment for our residents by developing innovative and creative occupational therapy programs that document participation and provide a means for ongoing evaluation. Program development also includes inservice training sessions to explain the roles and objectives of the OT programs for the various patients. The system involves the development of four stages: program planning, development of a written plan, implementation of the program, and evaluation of the program.

Program planning is a screening of the residents to assess their needs and interests. It includes their past and current interests, their social skills and present psychological functioning levels. This information is then compiled to identify the number of residents with the same needs, to decide which needs seem most critical, and to determine whether the COTA staff can provide a program to meet those needs. Appropriate activities are then selected to meet those needs.

The next step is the development of a written plan. It also includes the goals, the objectives, the modalities being used, and a plan of implementation. The third step is implementation of the program, which consists of informing the multidisciplinary team about the new program. Trial groups are conducted during this time ranging from one month to three months. The fourth stage of program development is the program evaluation process, which consists of a thorough review of all individual steps.

Compiling and documenting this information, offers the COTA staff the opportunity to develop new ideas and to try new techniques. Through this system we provide high quality therapeutic programs that increase our professional image in activity departments in long-term care facilities.

Bobbie Groth, COTA;
Julie Toppson, COTA[23]
Excerpts from COTA Concerns column, "Occupational Therapy News," April 1983.

SUGGESTIONS

1. Make a list of your positive and negative impressions about the aged.
2. Call your local office on Aging for information covering facts and activities.
3. Talk with aged persons. How are they different? How are they the same?
4. Go to an open house or special event at a nursing home. How did the residents react to you? How did their reactions make you feel?
5. Participate in conducting an activity at a Senior Center. Note the levels of interest and learning among the members.
6. Observe older individuals as you walk down the street. What characteristics make you classify a person as old?
7. Write your congressional representative for flyers covering current legislation effecting the aged.
8. Assist an occupational therapy assistant with a program for the aged. What does the OTA like about the job? What problems does it present? How often do the COTA and the OTR meet?
9. Contact the American Occupational Therapy Association for free recruitment literature emphasizing occupational therapy with the aged and where

you might see the AOTA film, "And When You Grow Old." Ask about obtaining the booklet, "Growing Old."

10. Find out about the many different types of programs servicing the aged in your community, such as home care services, clinics, community centers, mental health programs, hospitals, Meals on Wheels units, homes for the aged, retirement classes, etc. In which is occupational therapy already offered? How might occupational therapy be helpful where it does not yet exist?

READING OBJECTIVES

1. State the usual criteria for identifying a person as aged.
2. Discuss why both the physical and psychosocial components of an occupational therapy assistant curriculum are important for work with the aged.
3. Name and compare the two major types of programs in which an occupational therapy assistant would work with the aged.
4. Give examples of settings and occupational therapy services with the aged.

REFERENCES

[21]Davis L: Update-ROTE Project, Gerontology Special Interest Section, Newsletter, Vol. 7 No. 3, 1984.

[22]Phillipe N, Walker M: COTA and OTR Treatment Team in Schools. Occupational Therapy News. October, 1984.

[23]Groth B, Toppon J: Improving the Image of the COTA in Therapeutic Activity Programming. OT Newspaper, April, 1983.

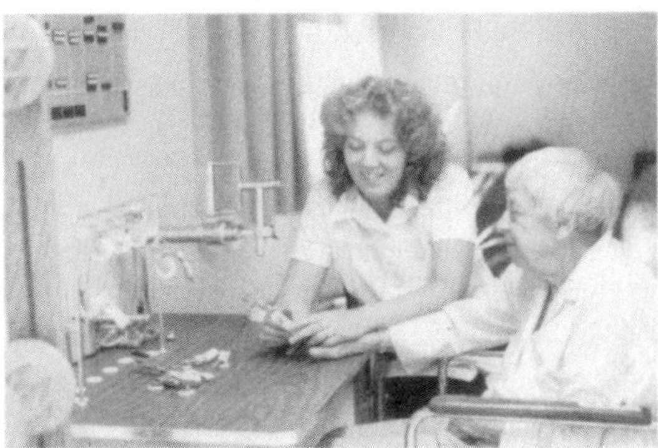

Figure 6-1: Sensitivity to the client's needs and feelings is important while positioning fingers in an exerciser.

CHAPTER 7

THE OCCUPATIONAL THERAPY ASSISTANT WORKS WITH CHILDREN

THE OCCUPATIONAL THERAPY ASSISTANT TREATS CHILDREN

What Kind of Children Need Occupational Therapy?

A large group of children being served by OTAs are those with cerebral palsy. These children often have multiple handicaps as a result of brain damage before, during or soon after birth. Occupational Therapy can be used to treat children with other defects and diseases found at birth as well (such as amputations and spina bifida). Children who have suffered from illnesses or injuries (for example, a fractured arm) may benefit from therapy. Children who are hospitalized temporarily and children with progressive chronic diseases (such as muscular dystrophy) may receive occupational therapy. Children with emotional problems and limited learning disabilities may also benefit from occupational therapy. OT programs may be designed for specialty groups such as autistic children or the blind or deaf as well.

Where Are They Found?

United Cerebral Palsy Centers throughout the country provide both residential and day treatment programs as do other specially designed centers. Hospital pediatric departments usually treat children for short stays. Chronic disease hospitals or specialty hospitals often have long term children's units. Special schools and residences provide services for designated populations and public schools are now enrolling and identifying children with special needs. Day treatment centers may be designed especially for children and home care services are also available.

How Does the Occupational Therapy Assistant Train to Work With Children?

While enrolled in an occupational therapy assistant training program the student is required to take courses in normal growth and development. These courses are often called developmental psychology or child psychology. They will help the student to understand and anticipate expected behaviors and abilities of children. To learn the physical developmental process the student must take courses in human biology, anatomy and physiology.

The training program should also include content on (1) maternal and child health; (2) the diseases that particularly effect children such as transmittable diseases (e.g., measles) and congenital defects with which a child might be born; (3) therapeutic activities that are particularly appropriate for children such as educational toys and developmental playthings as shown in Figure 7-1; (4) the value of play; (5) approaches to planning and leading groups; (6) goals and practices of occupational therapy with children; (7) responsibilities of other members of the treatment team; (8) therapeutic use of self; (9) appropriate techniques for self care skills at different age levels and for specific disabilities; and (10) carrying out stimulation of senses activities under supervision.

Trends and Opportunities

As a result of legislation mandating public schools to provide for the special needs of all children, an increasing number of occupational therapy assistants are being hired to work in schools in many sections of the country. Depending on individual state and local hiring practices occupational therapy assistants may be carrying out similar therapeutic approaches but may be given different titles. Training programs are being offered to experienced occupational therapy assistants who wish to specialize in this area. Occupational therapy assistants work in rehabilitation centers, schools, specialized treatment units (as with the blind/deaf), general hospital pediatric departments, chronic disease hospitals, children's mental health programs, residences, group homes and in home care. Increasing attention is being paid to pre-school and infant stimulation programs.

OCCUPATIONAL THERAPY ASSISTANTS IN PRACTICE

Occupational therapy assistants working in pediatrics may find themselves dealing with patients with a wide range of problems from the basically well population to the severely handicapped. Occupational therapy services have been in particularly great demand at two ends of the spectrum. An increasing number of occupational therapy assistants are being hired by school systems (particularly in the midwest) to work with learning disabled children. Another area in which an increasing number of occupational therapy assistants are being hired is in the expanding number of community based settings for the multiple handicapped. Examples of occupational therapy assistants working with children follow.

Community Autism Program

Linda realizes that her position in this program as an occupational therapy assistant working exclusively with autistic children is considered very demanding but feels that she is meeting an important need. Since it is primarily an after school, vacation period and summer program she knows that she can commit herself to the responsibility for short periods at a time. Linda is one of three staff members assigned to the group of autistic children in her classroom. She supervises a treatment aide and in turn reports to the occupational therapist. But most of the time they are all involved in direct supervision, interaction and handling of specific clients. The clients need constant observation, so one staff member has to cover when another has to follow or accompany one of the clients out of the room.

Linda is aware that the program is geared to help not only the autistic children themselves but their families as well. The families get some relief while the children are with Linda and they can learn from her and other staff how best to deal with certain behaviors the child is exhibiting. Therefore, Linda always arranges to see and speak with family members about each child, and reports new developments not only to the treatment team but to the family as well. Linda is prepared to accept limited goals in areas such as reducing abusive behavior, increasing self care, achieving in a task, increasing attention time, and mastering socially acceptable ways of interacting. Treatment modalities must be shown only one at a time in a sparse setting to minimize distraction. If for example a ball is used, Linda makes sure that it is used appropriately for play, provides structure and consistency and is ready to remove it if it is used inappropriately or attention wanes after a few minutes. Linda must be constantly ready to change an activity.

Residential Treatment Facility

Debbie works in a live-in facility for 20 children. It is housed in a former mansion and looks no different from the rest of the neighborhood. Originally only children with unique emotional disorders were accepted at the home for research purposes. Now children are referred by schools, by community agencies and physicians. A day treatment program is offered as well.

Debbie is involved in a variety of programs. Examples are: pre-vocational skill training including learning to attend on time and carry out an assigned task in an expected time period; personal belongings care including making the bed and keeping clothes in order; fitness programs including participating appropriately in group games like shuffleboard and following the rules when bicycle riding or sledding on the grounds; and educational skill development including working with the teachers to develop better perceptual ability or concentration.

Although it sometimes seems that a child is "just playing" when with

Debbie, she is actually carrying out a specific program to meet therapeutic needs. The variety of activities she uses may meet prescribed skills development through sports, mental activities, expressive arts, or promote leisure skills through hobbies and family related involvement. The goal might be to increase or develop basic functional skills, for example, to develop conversational ability in an 8 year old withdrawn boy she had him join a small group game and wrote and worked toward the specific goal of "the child will interact for 10 minutes with others."

Public School

Murry works as a paraprofessional in a public school which has a special floor for disabled students. Each day he and the occupational therapist greet the children as they come in since their day begins with taking off their outer clothing before going to classes. This provides a realistic opportunity for the occupational therapy assistant, Murry, to train disabled students to handle dressing more independently to the best of their abilities. A similar treatment approach is used at the end of the day when the students get ready to go home. The occupational therapy staff including Murry, assist them with their clothing while training them in techniques such as putting on a coat while sitting in a wheelchair or handling boots, gloves and scarves in spite of uncoordinated movements. During the day the occupational therapy routine is based on the needs of individual students. Murry is involved in making wheelchair adaptations including padding for the skin of sensitive students. One of his patients was a newly disabled 10 year old boy confined to a wheelchair as a result of a fall from a roof. Not only did he have to learn to compensate for his physical limitations, but he also needed to build up his self-esteem. Murry learned that the boy had enjoyed playing basketball prior to his accident, but had assumed that it would not be possible for him to play again. Considering individual needs led Murry to install a basketball hoop on the wall in the occupational therapy area. Then while shooting baskets the child could receive therapy for both his physical and emotional needs; he was strengthening his arms which he will have to depend on, and he was enjoying a sense of accomplishment and learning a potential activity for socialization with others. Wheelchair basketball is even a competitive sport.

The occupational therapy staff works very closely with other therapeutic staff. Sometimes Murry works jointly with the speech therapist and physical therapist with a child on the mat. The focus for the team might be developing the child's ability to roll over.

Developmental Institute

Lana is a COTA in a large institute for the multiple handicapped where she has gained special knowledge in oral facilitation (e.g., promoting proper swallowing) and designing adaptive wheelchairs. Lana usually attends a training workshop at least once a year to further her knowledge. When a patient's treatment program is established Lana may handle part of the program; the other part might be carried out by other staff.

Lana's day consists of carrying out treatments such as a meal time program, oral facilitation program, sensory stimulation therapy, or a developmental program. Part of her day is spent assisting a wheelchair team and helping to make decisions about adapting wheelchairs. She also orders any wheelchair parts that are needed. She may do a screening, ADL evaluation, or special evaluation. She also spends part of her day supervising two OT technicians.

The OT department consists of a director (a registered occupational therapist) and three other OTRs, four COTAs, five OT technicians and two therapeutic equipment specialists for the wheelchair shop. The OT program services community clients for evaluations and home programs. Each person in the department may carry out from six to thirteen treatments each day. At 7:30 a.m. Lana goes to a cottage and feeds a 5 year old boy his breakfast while using techniques to encourage proper use of his mouth and hands for eating. He is developing chewing and lip closure. She administers oral facilitation by stroking and manipulating his chin, cheeks, lips and tongue prior to his meal, and then feeds him.

Lana has another patient who ambulates unsteadily and lacks coordination. The patient's program consists of a variety of vestibular (balance) and tactile (touch) activities. The patient is unable to rock laterally (from side to side). If Lana can get her to accomplish this, she will have greater awareness of herself in space and be better able to handle self tasks.

Cerebral Palsy Center

Betty is a COTA who works in a center for children with cerebral palsy, a congenital condition resulting from brain damage. One of Betty's patients was a nine year old girl with limited muscle control. Betty saw the girl twice a week for a period of half an hour each visit. The child was using sanding blocks to make a project from wood. Betty tried to encourage any two hand activities, including having the girl move herself on a skate board. This was an excellent activity for the patient because it increased full range of motion and strength in both arms, built endurance and increased the child's attention span. It also helped her build self-esteem when the child saw how far she could travel alone. Betty reminded her to keep her fingers and hands straight. The child also played with a game called Lite-Brite (which is similar to putting pegs in a board). This helped with fine motor coordination, eye-hand coordination, and also provided for perceptual training. All of these activities helped the child to handle her daily self-care needs and learning objectives.

In treatment of children occupational therapy assistants usually work with one child at a time. Toys are frequently used therapeutically to promote physical, psychological and other goals directed toward the specific needs of the child. Stringing beads involves both perception and coordination and can be graded from larger to smaller sized beads as improvement is seen (Figure 7-1).

Hospital

Donna chose to work in the hospital because of the variety of patients and the fast-paced atmosphere. She learned that occupational therapy has many different functions in this setting. She assists the occupational therapist in making splints for children with burns so that when their skin heals joints will still have full mobility. She participates in early case finding helping to identify high risk patients soon after their birth and following through with approaches to stimulate their senses, particularly of hearing and seeing. She also deals with children hospitalized for surgery or long-term cancer treatment providing ways for them to express their feelings and cope with pain and separation. She even provides some services to the small 12 bed children's psychiatric unit where she leads activity groups directed toward such goals as increasing self esteem, developing social skills, increasing concentration and accepting and carrying out responsibilities. In addition to working directly with patients as assigned by the occupational therapist, Donna is also responsible for ordering and maintaining supplies and for supervising a volunteer who assists in setting up projects and providing activities.

Donna finds that she must have puzzles and items such as stacking toys available for the therapist who supervises the developmental program for preschoolers.

Children's Rehabilitation Unit

Lori likes the colorful atmosphere and the dedicated staff on the unit. Although the unit will take children as young as 3 months, the majority of its patients are between 5 and 8 years old. One of Lori's patients had muscular dystrophy, a disease in which the muscles get progressively weaker. Lori worked with him to maintain his strength and keep his joints mobile since he was sometimes too weak to move them himself. She showed him energy saving ways of taking care of himself as well. During the lunch hour Lori and the rest of the staff worked on a one to one basis with patients. At that time Lori arranged for a sling to support her patient's arm so that he could bring food to his mouth. She also provided him with a lightweight "spork" (spoon/fork combination) so that he wouldn't have to change utensils.

Children's Psychiatric Center

Victor likes working with the small group of 12 children in the psychiatric center. However, he had not anticipated how difficult some of the therapeutic tasks might be. He has learned to provide structure for himself and the children, to realize that some goals take longer to accomplish, and that not all children respond to therapy in the same way. Although he generally works alone with one child, he also shares the leadership of a group and uses activities which require more than one adult (such as a parachute as shown in Figure 7-2).

The major areas he works toward with the children are: increasing verbalization, self-expression and social skills; decreasing atypical behaviors and mannerisms; increasing capacity for self-control; and increasing independence and ability to make decisions. Primarily he uses crafts, games and group projects such as making decorations for a party.

Burn and Trauma Center

Rebecca was fortunate to have a supervising occupational therapist who saw her skills and potential and worked with her to develop her expertise in splinting, special devices and approaches for severely injured children. Through practice and initial guidance Rebecca has become experienced with the many materials available and the important precautions to be considered. Rebecca treats patients with a wide range of ailments. One child had broken a wrist as a result of a fall. Rebecca had the child work at a device made from a shovel handle which encourages the child to twist the wrist to get full motion. Another child was burned when he tipped over a pot of hot water. Rebecca positioned devices for him to keep motion in the joints while his skin is healing. Rebecca also works with a child in a coma as a result of an automobile accident. Rebecca provides stimulation to all senses and passive movement for the child.

Rebecca must be sensitive to the needs of both the children and parents through the long course of treatment. She continues to consult with her supervisor and other staff to be sure she is meeting overall team goals.

IN THE WORDS OF OCCUPATIONAL THERAPY ASSISTANTS

I became interested in occupational therapy by working in a classroom as an aide in a school for physically handicapped children. I enjoyed the challenge through OT of finding ways of allowing the handicapped to function as normally as possible. In particular I was impressed with use of Cybertype which was at that time being tried under a Federal grant by our school. Several students were learning to type with their feet.

As the only COTA in the Grand Rapids School System I was in the position of setting the criteria and uses for possible future COTAs. I work under a part time OTR, and the position was more or less created for me.

My responsibilities include teaching pre-vocational classes and typing using adaptive equipment such as mouth stick head pointers, encouraging leisure skills, making adaptive equipment or advising or helping teachers with the use of it, record keeping, and testing and evaluating students.

For those considering a career as an occupational therapy assistant I suggest that you shadow a COTA for a week to see if this is really what you want.

Frances Miller, COTA
Ottawa Hills High School
Physically & Otherwise Health Impaired Center
Grand Rapids, Michigan

When in college, we were told to investigate each job situation and use ourselves and our skills accordingly. In my current position as a teacher assistant there are about 20 autistic children and adolescents in 3 classrooms with 10 staff. My class is extremely disturbed. We work on sitting, listening and learning skills. Eye contact and performing simple commands along with language development are our main emphasis. My emphasis is self care, such as zipping, buttoning, dressing and brushing teeth. I very much see a place for vestibular and tactile stimulation but I am the only person trained in occupational therapy and find it difficult to plan a sensorimotor program myself.

The guidelines I use are: Be resourceful, imaginative and suggestive—meaning voicing my ideas.

Johanna Breault, COTA
Quimby Regional Cooperative
School for Seriously Disturbed Youth
Worcester, Massachusetts

SUGGESTIONS

1. Volunteer your services with hospitalized children.
2. Note how children react to music, dance, play and other activities.
3. Observe an occupational therapy program for a child or group of children. What kind of activities are used?
4. Visit an occupational therapy pediatrics department. What kind of equipment is visible? What level of training has the staff had? Are the children treated on a "one to one" basis or does one staff member work with more than one child at a time?
5. Look through job listings for occupational therapy personnel. Notice the types of settings serving children and the salaries offered.

READING OBJECTIVES

1. Identify the treatment setting most rapidly expanding as the primary site for occupational therapy services with children.
2. List the subjects which best prepare the occupational therapy assistant for work with children.
3. Discuss the job opportunities in this area of practice.
4. Give examples of the kinds of children treated by occupational therapy assistants and the therapeutic goals established.

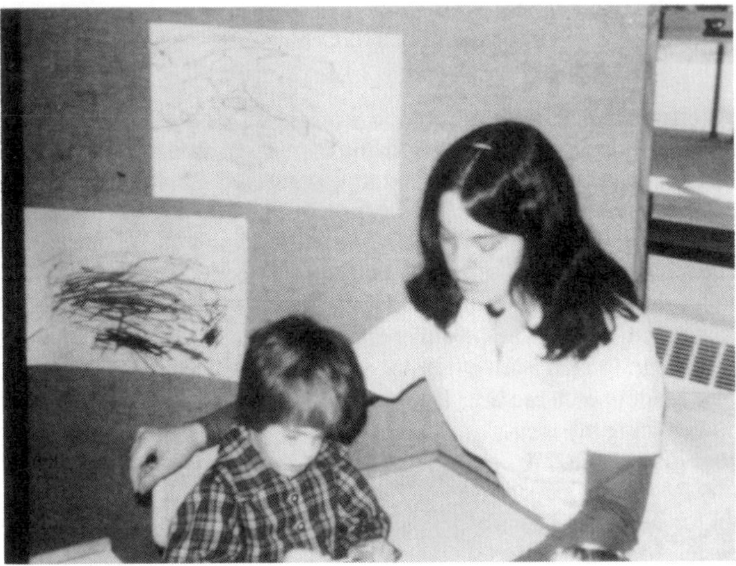

Figure 7-1: The occupational therapy assistant works closely with the child to assure that the activity is done appropriately to meet the therapeutic goal.

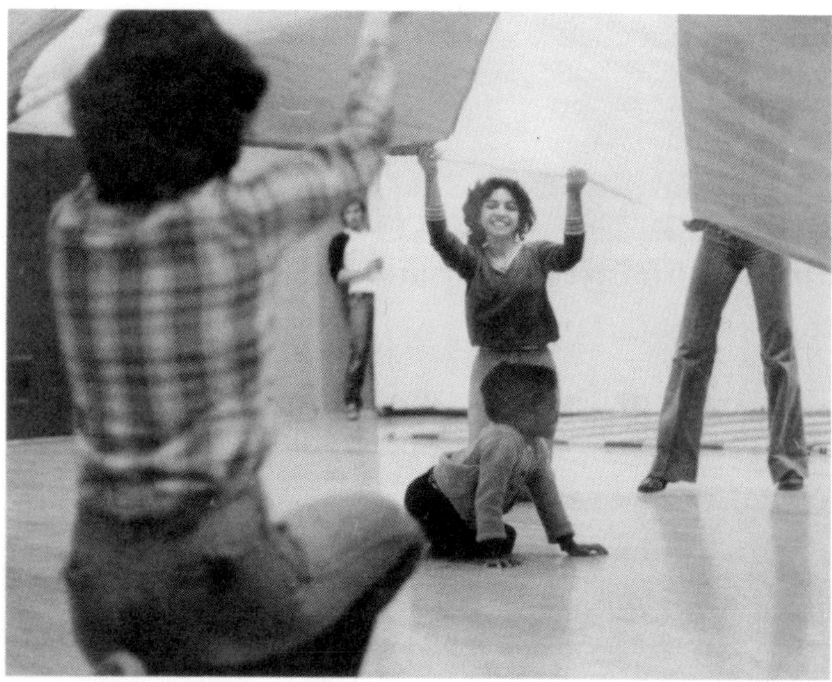

Figure 7-2: A parachute is used by an occupational therapy assistant as a therapeutic activity to promote sensory and perceptual awareness, to encourage particular physical movements and to stimulate interaction with others.

CHAPTER 8

THE OCCUPATIONAL THERAPY ASSISTANT WORKS IN THE AREA OF DEVELOPMENTAL DYSFUNCTION

DEVELOPMENTAL DYSFUNCTION—AN IMPORTANT AREA FOR THE OCCUPATIONAL THERAPY ASSISTANT

Populations

Persons who have delayed development, who have learning disorders and who are mentally retarded are often classified as developmentally disabled. Those with cerebral palsy and autism are often included in developmental centers as well as retarded adults. Those who are mentally retarded may be older in years but younger in behavior and thought and may have physical as well as mental delays.

Opportunities

There is a growing demand for occupational therapy assistants to work in the area of developmental dysfunction. For many years those designated as retarded were serviced primarily in large state institutions where their living needs were provided. Health and legislative planning have led to the establishment of smaller facilities within residential communities. This encourages and provides an opportunity for the family to become involved and interested in the client's treatment and progress. More staff have been hired to provide intensive therapy, in many ways recognizing the potential for growth and development and the learning of acceptable behaviors which may enable such a person to function to his maximum level.

In these new developmental centers increased numbers of professional staff provide active intervention, and each client is expected to reach his maximum potential. A positive approach is established based on the identified needs and goals of each client.

In the course of treatment a series of progressive steps is established. The achievement of set goals is designated as measured progress. The ability of the patient to repeat and accomplish them in an appropriate time period is also important. The role of occupational therapy in this area is quite significant since the emphasis is on improving functional living skills. Increasing numbers of occupational therapy assistants are being recruited for this specialty area, since once the client has been evaluated and goals established, the OTA is particularly equipped to assure the carrying out of the repetitive treatment program and record the achievement of each interim goal.

Preparation

To work with the developmentally impaired it is important to know both the psychological and physical aspects of normal growth and development. Causes of retardation are also learned. The student learns how persons are classified as mildly, severely or profoundly retarded and how to record observations and distinguish between observations and interpretations. Information about what testing procedures are used and how they are administrated and graded is made available. It is important to consider the positive and negative aspects of labeling, testing, institutionalization, and various approaches to treatment and handling of the retarded. The student must be aware of personal values and professional reactions to such individuals. Society may reflect negative attitudes toward the retarded that are not relevant and may interfere with the student's ability to treat such patients.

Since traditional crafts and activities geared toward the chronological age of a patient may not be appropriate for his or her mental age, modifications and flexibility in treatment are important. The student must learn to follow appropriate goals for the level of the patient. Even "simple" tasks may have to be projected over a long time period and will need to be broken down into step-by-step patterns to be realistically achieved. Repetition is also crucial for behavior change. Structure and consistency will have to be provided by the assistant. And, finally the student will learn to make appropriate adapted equipment and to use such assistive techniques as hand-over-hand (the therapist's hand guiding the client's hand) in order to teach patients eating.

OCCUPATIONAL THERAPY ASSISTANTS ON THE JOB

In large developmental centers some OTAs have chosen to specialize in particular areas such as the making of adaptive equipment or assistive devices.

Adapted Equipment Unit

Larry, while in OTA school, enjoyed woodworking and designing unique specialized equipment. He was hired by the occupational therapy department in a state supported developmental center to construct devices and equipment which would enable the clients to increase their functional abilities and care for themselves more independently. Examples of the items he made include a high back for a chair, a separator to keep legs from closing like a pair of scissors, and rear view mirrors for wheelchairs of children who only have the ability to push backwards.

Community Based Developmental Center

Justine is not only the only certified occupational therapy assistant in her development center but also the only full time person in the occupational therapy department. The registered occupational therapist makes weekly evaluations of patients and plans and makes changes in their treatment where indicated. Most of Justine's patients are severely or profoundly retarded young children. She works in a newly designed large occupational therapy room with brightly painted equipment and wall murals, low child-size tables and chairs, blocks and toys, standing mirrors, various sized balls and climbing equipment. Using all this equipment, Justine enables her patients to reach, grasp, pinch, coordinate their movements and manipulate appropriately in response to what their eyes see and their minds perceive should be done.

At lunchtime, Justine and other professional staff, work with the children while they eat, each therapist working in his or her areas of expertise. The speech therapist assists one child in learning to suck and swallow, movements that are important for speech as well as eating. At the other end of the table, Justine enables a 6 year old to pick up the appropriate utensil, get food onto it and bend his arm so that the food will go to his mouth without spilling. To accomplish this Justine selected and made for the child a swivel spoon with a thick bent handle and a plate guard.

Day Program

Myrna is an occupational therapy assistant in a day center. Most of her clients live at home or in group homes and arrive by bus each day for both learning and therapy sessions. They are ages 13–15 and grouped according to their level of functioning. When she treats the high functioning group, she is able to use a variety of crafts and games and encourages socialization. With another group she concentrates on prevocational tasks involving checking in, counting tokens or stacking boxes in a store like setting.

One of her clients has a visual problem in addition to developmental delay and physical limitations. She works with him on an individual basis and in the socialization group. She assists him in catching a large ball to encourage use of both hands, to tilt his chin so that he can swallow more easily, and gently helps him to extend his fingers as he finger paints. In teaching him to button, Myrna first used a board fitted with large buttons and loops on material. She taught him the concept of going "through." On the board he could visualize the button going through. He then proceeded to a board with regular size buttons which was brightly colored so that the buttons could be easily seen. After mastering that he tried large buttons on himself and finally smaller ones.

Myrna also leads a group with the speech therapist. The group discusses the goals and problems of improving their independent living skills with regard to returning home or to a group home. They also discuss attitudes toward disability, their attitudes toward themselves and their own body image.

Group Home

One of Janet's patients is assigned to the occupational therapy unit to improve grooming habits and work on dressing techniques. He is mildly retarded, 23 years old, with physical malformations. He has no control of his right hand and he wears an orthopedic shoe and moves with a cane. Janet demonstrated and taught him washing approaches and ways to assist in dressing. These included special techniques for putting a shirt over his head and a sponge devise which holds the soap and allows him to wash himself.

Private Hospital

Richard chose to work in a new developmental center, a private hospital, in his own community. He enjoyed the opportunity to walk to work and felt he could relate to those who were of the same background as himself. The developmental center uses a system of precise recording of both long and short-term goals. Specific tasks were introduced to accomplish these goals, and the patient's progress as a result of the occupational therapy program was observed and recorded. Although it might take a long time for a patient to accomplish the goal, of drinking from a cup for instance, by recording all steps involved, progress can be observed and noted. A breakdown of steps might be as follows: recognize the glass, reach for it, lift it, bring it to the mouth, and drink.

Richard works closely with his supervisor, the registered occupational therapist who assigns patients to him, outlines goals, and determines when program changes should be made. She observes him during the week and meets with him. Richard attends the occupational therapy staff meetings, and the rehabilitation team meeting and is responsible for his own unit providing occupational therapy for all of the children who need it in the ward to which he was assigned. He has a large treatment room and two aides to assist him. Most of his contact with the children in his assigned unit is on a one-to-one basis.

One of his patients was a 12 year old boy profoundly retarded who was about the same size as a normal 3 year old. The child had been living in a large state institution before the new community developmental center was established. Richard first worked with him on activities that might lead to his being able to do basic functions independently. To help the child improve balance a very large (3 ft. diameter) inflated ball was used in treatment. Richard had the child balance on the ball while an aide showed him a special toy. The goal was for the child to reach for the toy while still maintaining balance on the ball.

Sheltered Workshop

Lisa works with older teenagers and adults in a workshop which provides employment for retarded individuals who cannot work in a competitive work situation usually because they need more time to complete the work task. A regular work setting must meet the government minimum wage per hour. A sheltered workshop is allowed to pay on a piece work basis. In other words if the "normal" individual completes, for example, 10 packages each hour, then the client or worker in the sheltered workshop would get one tenth (1/10) of the minimum wage per hour for each package completed. Lisa's responsibilities include helping to determine the "norms" (how many items the fully capable worker would do per hour).

School

Deborah likes the short day that her school job as an occupational therapy assistant allows. Another "benefit" she finds in this setting is that much less record keeping is required. Although she participates in the individual plan required for each student, she does not have to meet the continuous need for written records generally required in health care facilities. Therefore, Deborah has more time to spend in direct patient contact. She sees students, as they arrive, showing them how to take off their outer garments, taking them out of classes to work on perception and motor skills, helping at lunch to improve self feeding, and involving them in groups to promote social and vocational skills. Some of the therapeutic approaches Deborah uses include puzzles, scooters, short handled eating utensils, and sorting tasks.

Child Development Program

Margaret is an experienced occupational therapy assistant who works in a child development program. She had a 7 year old patient who was profoundly mentally retarded. The patient had difficulties with movement and control in both his arms and legs. Margaret involved him in a gross motor program using large movements to facilitate normal movement patterns and to enable the patient to engage more effectively in fine motor activities and achieve higher developmental levels. His OT program included activities on a mat and use of a large therapeutic ball and a scooter board. In each of the activities two people were needed to accomplish the goals. Therefore Margaret supervised an aide who assisted her. Margaret observed that while the patient lay on top of the 4 ft. diameter ball and tried to maintain his balance, his head extension relaxed and he learned to protect his limbs. His head control and increase of muscle tone were improved by the use of the scooter board. For the patient's safety, he was strapped on the scooter board and instructed to keep his hands away from the wheels as he moved himself along with a crawling motion. Margaret recorded all details to determine progress. She noted that the patient lifted his head from the scooter board twice when going forward and three times going backwards.

Margaret applied touch and movement stimulation to his body, arms and legs and properly positioned him lying face down and on his side. Using an air mattress helped to stimulate tactile (touch) sensations. Margaret has learned to set precise limited goals and to adjust her expectations accordingly to meet the needs of her patients and to feel needed as well.

IN THE WORDS OF AN OCCUPATIONAL THERAPY ASSISTANT

Initially, I came to the school as a fieldwork student. A teaching position became available and I was offered the job and accepted. There seemed to be a need for more flexibility and creativity...for more coordination and communication between the teachers, therapists and parents. The OTR and I developed group sessions with the school parent group that often considered topics relevant to the parents' concerns or priorities. The parents responded to the coordinated treatment approach, sought more active involvement and provided information on their children's behavior and performance in the home environment. I realized that some of these combined treatment program goals could be met in various community programs and asked the parents to consider treatment environments other than the school and the home. I began taking my class to the park once a week for a gymnastic-swimming program. During these sessions I provided task analysis of community activities and this further facilitated treatment carry over in the home. Unfortunately, I was forced to leave the school because physical tolerance for full time work was impaired due to injuries sustained in a car accident. The parents decided to employ me and continue our program. I now work with the parents and children in their homes.

I maintain contact with the professionals at the school and now adapt treatment programs and activities to the home settings. I also provide suggestions to the parents on constructive use of leisure time with their children. The use of community programs has expanded.

It has been very rewarding for me to have been instrumental in improving communication between the school and the parents. The children work as a group; the parents work as a group; the staff has become a group. The result is one large group working for the benefit of these children.[24]
Diane Schmidt, COTA
New Horizon Center
for the Developmentally Disabled
Chicago, IL

TRENDS AND OPPORTUNITIES

Developmental Dysfunction is one of the fastest growing areas for the occupational therapy assistant. Changing legislation and community interest have led to dynamic new programs for those with developmental problems including learning dysfunction, retardation and various neurological disorders grouped in the category. Large state facilities are being replaced by smaller community based units. Those with developmental dysfunction are being mainstreamed into classrooms which can provide "the least restrictive environment."

There is an increasing emphasis on measurable objectives. Goals are defined precisely and achievement noted. As progress is observed to be possible for this population there is an additional demand for therapy personnel to carry out the programs that lead to progress. These include self care activities and vocational readiness programs such as that shown in Figure 8-1.

Occupational therapy assistants today work with the developmentally disabled on such daily living tasks as handling money, travel training and self care (Figure 8-1). This is to enable them to prepare for community living, an increasing emphasis in this field.

SUGGESTIONS

1. Contact your local associations for the mentally retarded.
2. Collect and read available literature.
3. Find out where treatment centers for developmental dysfunction are located and whether occupational therapy is available.
4. Visit a developmental center.
   a. Observe the kinds of play and treatment materials available and the creative activities used.
   b. Ask what short-term and long-term occupational therapy goals have been established for a selected individual receiving occupational therapy services.

c. Try to look at a treatment goal form. Note the various categories including the specific task the client must achieve, the number of repetitions to be completed and the amount of time expected for its achievement.

READING OBJECTIVES

1. Identify the population described as developmentally disabled.
2. Discuss the changes occurring in this field of practice.
3. List subjects which prepare the occupational therapy assistant for work with the developmentally disabled.
4. Give examples of settings for this population and the kind of occupational therapy provided.

REFERENCES

[24]Excerpted from COTA Role in School Programs. Occupational Therapy News, 1984.

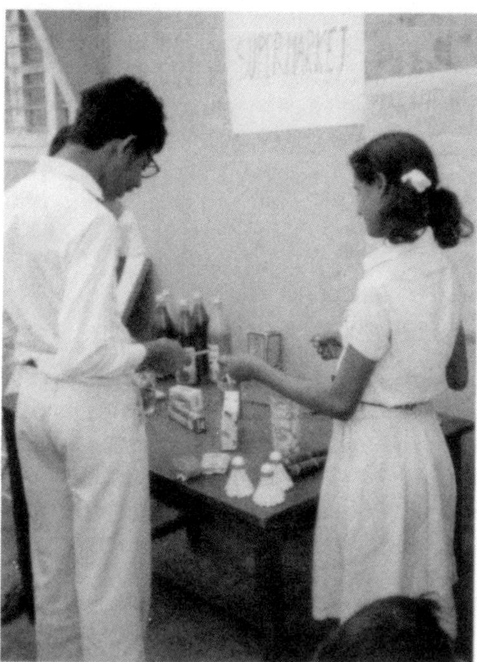

Figure 8-1: Here mentally retarded adolescents are trained to handle shopping independently.

CHAPTER 9

THE OCCUPATIONAL THERAPY ASSISTANT WORKS IN MENTAL HEALTH

MENTAL HEALTH: AN IMPORTANT AREA FOR THE OCCUPATIONAL THERAPY ASSISTANT

What is Meant by Mental Illness?

Everyday we face routine tasks, challenges, new experiences and problems. We generally adjust to the changing demands of our day and respond appropriately to each situation. Mental health programs serve those individuals who have difficulties with everyday activities, in understanding how they are to proceed, in responding or reacting to expectations and in coping with changes. Such people may not have the resiliency to recover after stress or disturbance.

Clients participating in mental health programs include those who cannot cope with a recent crisis, drug abusers, alcoholics, those with specific problems such as phobias or anorexia, those who need a structured environment—perhaps only temporarily, severely depressed individuals, those who cannot carry out daily activities, abnormally excited persons, and those with psychotic episodes or long-term disorders such as schizophrenia.

Where are the Mentally Ill?

The largest facilities for the mentally ill are usually state psychiatric hospitals or private centers which often have smaller units located on the same grounds or in the community. Community based day hospitals or day treatment centers may be found in store fronts, as part of general community centers or in their own free standing facilities. They generally focus on a variety of activity programs during the day with special therapy or medication offered where indicated. Large general hospitals often have a small psychiatric unit. Residential or day treatment centers for special populations are available. Partial hospitalization programs exist independently or within broader institutions. Single room occupancy hotels or shelters often have aftercare clinics. Other follow-up services for those discharged from psychiatric hospitals include adult homes, group homes and day programs sponsored by non-profit agencies.

How Does the Occupational Therapy Assistant Prepare for a Job in Mental Health?

Approved occupational therapy assistant training programs include courses in: general and developmental psychology, group dynamics or group processes, abnormal psychology or psychiatric conditions, occupational therapy media & skills or applications & techniques, occupational therapy theory & practice in mental health or psychosocial dysfunction, and fieldwork in psychiatry. Mary Beth Early's *Mental Health Concepts for the Occupational Therapy Assistant*, published by Raven Press, is a newly used textbook.

The above courses are the primary preparation for the area of mental health. It must be remembered, however, that one of the concepts taught in occupational therapy training programs is that the occupational therapy assistant treats the individual as a whole. That is why the student is offered a general program so that the knowledge can be integrated and used where and when needed. An important concept to learn is "Therapeutic Use of Self." It implies that the assistant's manner of dealing with the client also serves as a therapeutic agent when used appropriately. The occupational therapy assistant can encourage or discourage, foster dependence or independence and help to motivate the patients or clients. Full appreciation for this skill often does not develop until field work is experienced.

In What Areas Can Occupational Therapy Help?

The occupational therapy assistant working in mental health may facilitate improvement in a variety of areas:

Activities of Daily Living	Clients referred for occupational therapy may not be able to carry out appropriate self care tasks, work responsibilities or participate in leisure activities.
Cognition	Clients may have difficulties in comprehension, communication, problem solving, integration of time management, conceptualization, learning, judgment, or orientation to time and place or person.
Self Identity & Concept	The client may not be able to separate self needs and expectations from those of others, identify areas of self competency and limitation, accept responsibility for self, perceive sexuality of self, have self respect, have appropriate body image, view self as being able to influence events. The patient/client may not have the necessary coping skills such as holding back aggressive impulses, sublimating urges, finding ways to satisfy own

	needs, tolerating frustration and anxiety (disappointments), experiencing gratification and controlling impulses.
Social Interpersonal Skills	Clients may need to develop their abilities in relationships to peers, subordinates and authority figures. This may include trust, respect, or warmth in perceiving and responding to needs and feelings of others, engaging in and sustaining independent relationships, and communicating feelings.
Group Interactional Skills	The client may need to develop performance tasks in the presence of others, such as sharing responsibilities with others, cooperating and competing with others, fulfilling a variety of group membership roles, expressing leadership skills, perceiving and responding to needs of group members.
Work Skills	The client may need to improve work habits including attendance or punctuality as well as specific skills related to the handling of job related tasks and materials.

OPPORTUNITIES AND TRENDS

Occupational therapy assistants are being hired increasingly in residential and day treatment centers in the community. OTAs are often given responsibility for conducting group activities in a variety of life skills or interest areas.

In both government and private psychiatric centers, occupational therapy assistants may be responsible for managing daily schedules for persons in particular treatment units, for providing training programs in self care and for preparing patients to return to home and work responsibilities. There are many job openings for occupational therapy assistants in mental health settings and opportunities for advancement into supervisory positions are available.

The area of mental health includes a variety of psychosocial dysfunctions. Occupational therapy assistants working in substance abuse programs, shelters and stress reduction are able to build on their basic training skills and become involved in the many emerging health issues in this area of practice. Examples of specific *treatment settings* follow.

Community Mental Health Center

Jennifer, a COTA in a mental health program, works primarily with group activities for clients who come into the center for the day. She designed a new group for some of the clients to learn appropriate use of leisure time. It provided an opportunity for creative expression. The group meets two hours and uses materials such as soap and potatoes to make prints on paper or cards. Jennifer uses therapeutic techniques including providing support or structure when needed, encouraging problem solving and group interaction. Inappropriate behavior or unexcused absences merits expulsion from the group. Thus stability is provided. Jennifer finds it a challenge to help the patients choose an artistic medium which meet both the therapeutic goals and budget and space restrictions of the program.

Examples of other groups Jennifer directs to meet therapeutic goals are: advertisement of self, where the participants each write an ad "selling" themselves; group meal preparation; the game of Charades; designing a traditional coat of arms; and creative arts constructions or group collage, where patients cut shapes from materials or paper and decide together where they will be glued to form a mural planned by the participants.

Adult Home

Yvette directs a unique occupational therapy program in a facility which primarily houses older adults who have been discharged from long-term psychiatric centers into a less intense setting in their own community. In addition to general activities programs, Yvette plans and supervises a workshop program where residents carry out tasks in a job-like atmosphere. They are required to arrive and leave on time and to be productive in completing work assignments during this scheduled placement. Approximately 18 residents attend each day. Projects range from simple collating or preparing mailings for community organizations and stapling to assembling items such as ball point pens.

Crisis Intervention Center

Pauline, a COTA who saw becoming an OT Assistant as a way to upgrade her career, works at a crisis intervention center. On a typical day she works with a number of patients. For example, Pauline was working on a puzzle with a 20 year old man, an activity to help him increase his concentration span to develop workable skills. Soon another patient joined the first. This meeting was arranged by Pauline to encourage interpersonal relationships. Pauline confronted the patient about inappropriate behavior. When he acted out, she set limits. She pointed out that originally she had him working on smaller puzzles with larger pieces. Because of his progress she introduced a more difficult puzzle in an effort to improve his frustration tolerance. The puzzle with more and smaller pieces was also used to explore his vocational aptitude with a structured and repetitive activity in an effort to prepare him for a post discharge rehabilitation program. Pauline pointed out that in this short term setting, puzzles which require varying levels of competence were chosen while a project such as wood working which could also have gradations (such as starting with an easy small task first) might have been chosen in a long term setting. This would have provided more opportunities to confront the client about inappropriate behavior and setting limits.

Pauline, who chose her career after her 3 children were grown, finds the psychiatric setting particularly interesting because she can be sensitive to the feelings of others as they communicate in words and gestures.

Patients come to the crisis intervention center on a voluntary basis. All of the 21 patients at the center attend occupational therapy where the approach is to deal with the immediate problem. The philosophy is based on the dynamics of milieu therapy in which the total environment is therapeutic.

Residence

Diane is the only COTA in a residence for persons who had been hospitalized for mental health problems in the past. Most of the clients are adolescents or young adults who still have difficulties in providing for their own daily needs. One of the residents was a 25 year old man who had been living at home with his parents while completing college. In helping to establish goals for carrying out occupational therapy, Diane participated in evaluating his sense of responsibility, self care, home care abilities, and academic skills. The focus of the program was on chores required to keep the residence functioning. Diane used these tasks in both the observations for the evaluation and in treatment.

In the area of work skills the client was observed cleaning the public rooms of the house and shopping for groceries. He tended to drift away and wasn't motivated to learn how to do the chores. His academic abilities were evaluated through conversations with him and by consulting with other staff. He was both intelligent and aware but did not connect his actions with their consequences and showed confusion at times. To determine his self care abilities, his general appearance, the manner in which he dresses, and his personal hygiene were observed. This was determined to be a problem area; his clothes were generally dirty and his whole appearance showed lack of care.

To determine the client's use of leisure time, he was observed during free time in the residence and interviewed. Much of his extra time was spent drinking or eating too much to relieve the boredom, isolation and loneliness that he often felt. His homemaking skills were observed through his participation in a cooking group with other residents. He lacked basic knowledge and was unwilling to work with others. To accomplish the goal of promoting independence, Diane assigned him to a cooking group and worked with him on an individual basis in chores and cleaning. She taught him to use a sponge mop including techniques such as wetting the sponge rather than the top. She provided positive feedback and got him to respond more. She gave him tasks and saw that they were done, such as sweeping the floor and cleaning the windows. She would interject comments such as, "I think it would be better if you used paper towels," or "Try to stay with it for a while." She encouraged him to take a messenger job and gave him information about the arrangements necessary.

Day Treatment Programs

Janice, Sandy and Jack work in different types of day treatment programs.

Janice works in a *day center* in a mental health program where clients not only have the opportunity to use a fast food counter in the lounge but to operate it as well. Janice, a COTA, as a member of the activity therapy staff, is responsible for the operation of the fast food service as a therapeutic group. It is called the commissary and is primarily for coffee breaks in the recreation room. It is used by both staff and patients as well as students from a nearby school. The commissary is operated by assigned clients on Monday, Wednesday, and Friday mornings. On Tuesdays, Janice leads the group in a discussion of plans for preparing meals for the week. On Wednesdays, part of the group goes shopping for the required food.

The therapeutic goals met include increased socialization; communication development; positive work habits including punctuality, good attendance and confidence in proper grooming; preparation for paid employment or volunteer work; development of a sense of belonging and usefulness; and high self esteem.

The activities to meet these goals include baking cakes, making coffee, serving customers breakfast and lunch, preparing meals and cooking. There are a clean up crew, servers, a set up crew, bakers, and coffee makers. Twice a week those assigned meet with an activity therapist to discuss progress, job possibilities and proper attire.

Janice is responsible for leading the discussion group, for handling problems that occur in the operation of the commissary, for playing the part of an employer, for documenting progress, for choosing discussion topics and for responding to clients regarding likes and dislikes. When a client develops good work habits, shows that he gets along well with others, can travel independently and has gained self esteem he is then discharged from the group and referred for a paid or unpaid regular job or position. Janice meets with her supervisor frequently to discuss these decisions and her responsibilities.

Sandy's role as an activities therapist in an *aftercare program* brings her in direct contact with a variety of persons who were formerly patients in psychiatric centers. One patient was admitted at age 30 after having received psychiatric treatment of various types since the age of six. After her most recent hospitalization, the patient was assigned to the aftercare activities therapy program. She participated in a clerical production group three times a week. Twice a week she attended a socialization group which aims at encouraging participants to start talking with one another and to take responsibility. The group takes trips every other week into the community. This is a therapeutic activity in itself and provides examples on how to use leisure time. Sometimes discussions are held, or at least attempted. Otherwise participants play Scrabble, checkers, cards, and other games.

One of Sandy's patients was a 28 year old client who lived with her husband and five children in a four room apartment shared with her sister and two other children. The patient was diagnosed as a chronic paranoid schizophrenic. Due to the medication she took, she suffered from blurred vision, aching muscles and constipation. She had been a methadone addict. She acted strangely at home, could not stay awake for long periods, and yelled about and to her dead sister. An occupational therapy program was designed to help the patient stay awake, to enable her to participate in activities on the ward, to reduce her restlessness, to increase her ability to tolerate frustration and to provide structure and stability which would help her to carry out simple daily chores upon her return home. The program included the patient's participation in activities that would require sitting and concentration. The amount of time and effort required was gradually increased. Her first projects were designed to provide almost immediate gratification, for example, tooling a design on metal foil and making belts out of leather. She began to make more challenging things and set her mind on constructing a rather complicated wooden bench. The bench tested her progress in tolerance of frustration since it was a step by step project, and she was not allowed to leave the OT workshop area until each step was completed.

At the *community outreach program* established by a settlement house, Jack, a COTA, worked with a man who was first hospitalized at the age of 19 with delusions of persecution and unpredictable behavior based on hallucinations. But these symptoms were not present when Jack began with the patient. However, he showed drowsiness and lethargic behavior which might be attributed to his medication. The patient tried to isolate himself physically and was unable to respond to questions. His speech and his judgment were impaired. He spoke of the settlement house as a club. In addition, at the age of 50, he had a number of other medical conditions particularly related to his heart and respiratory system.

Jack visited the client's apartment where he lives alone and from which he walks to the settlement house each day. Clothing and music records were strewn all over the apartment. This plus the fact that the patient's clothes showed dirt stains, indicated that the client should be assigned to the clothing care group in which patients participate in a full program of laundry activities including sorting, washing, drying, folding and ironing, if necessary.

Jack taught his patient each step of the project separately, reviewing and reinforcing previous steps. His client was also given very clear instructions.

Adolescent Treatment Center

Gladys chose to train as an OT assistant after having completed a degree in another area. She particularly appreciates the variety of employment opportunities in occupational therapy. Gladys can be observed in an activities therapy department in a psychiatric center where she works primarily with adolescents. She gets satisfaction from being able to start groups related to her own interest and skill and to be able to see the improvement in those she treats.

She leads a creative arts group which provides patients with an activity which facilitates coping effectively with situations in which maladaptive behavior—impulsivity, grandiosity, anger, denial and externalization—typically occur. In the group Gladys has patients who have had problems with acting on impulse, poor planning and problem solving behavior, poor judgment, being defiant of authority, being over compliant, inappropriate self assertiveness, and repetitive behavior.

Gladys must encourage group decision making and discussion, recommend the kind of art or craft and procedure that allows for self expression, introduce activities which require structure, use art materials which simulate feelings that can be expressed through the activity (i.e., working with clay, drawing, painting), and choose activities such as making posters, which involve the whole group.

The results of Gladys' creative arts group for the patients are improvement in dealing with others, increased confidence in self expression, increased tolerance of frustration, a sense of integrity, and improvement in the ability to help one's self.

Another group which Gladys leads is a weekly cooking group which includes 4 patients. At each meeting the group discusses what equipment is needed and the steps involved in preparing a simple food dish. The food is prepared by the group as a whole with each member required to participate in at least one step. While the prepared food is eaten, the group reviews the procedure and considers what was done well and what could be done differently next time. All participants then wash the dishes and utensils and clean the kitchen.

Through the activity, patients learn to plan and carry out a task in a logical sequence and to better manage their daily life. They also become familiarized with an environment similar to that in which they will prepare their own food upon return to the community. In addition they become more aware of their surroundings through stimulation of their senses, including the sense of taste. This activity also helps to relieve the fear of discharge and make patients less dependent on the hospital.

General Hospital

Marsha returned to school after having been a homemaker for several years. Her interest in working with people who may be neglected by others, coupled with a desire to find a "solid" occupation to provide for herself and her son, led her to occupational therapy.

Marsha works in a small psychiatric unit in a general hospital where there was a need for one of the OT staff to be available one weekend day. Marsha liked the idea of working on the weekend since she could have one day off during the week. The main purpose of the psychiatric unit is to help patients in a crisis to return to their earlier level of functioning through therapy. Marsha, as the COTA, works with a nurse as co-leader in a community group session. She also works with a group of patients in the OT room, along with the occupational therapist. A gardening group using house plants is one of the regular activities.

One of the features of the unit is one-to-one meetings whereby any staff member including the COTA, is designated as primary therapist for a particular client. The focus of Marsha's meetings with a patient could be on self care, participation, response to the assigned routine or an area of the patient's choosing. Marsha prepares a patient for discharge. In working with a female patient to improve grooming skills, Marsha teaches the client to wash her face using soap and water and to pat it dry. She then must choose the proper shade of makeup and apply it with light strokes. To develop the client's ability to rely on herself Marsha takes the client on trips to the bank to learn how to handle the necessary steps in caring for her own money. To prevent rehospitalization Marsha helps the client to structure her day's activities. The patient also explores potential opportunities for employment, trying various work skills and participating in pre-vocational training.

Psychiatric Hospital

Beverly, Ilene and Joe all work in different units of a large psychiatric hospital which often employs more than 10 occupational therapy assistants.

Beverly finds her work as a COTA in the *admitting* unit of the suburban psychiatric center quite interesting, because there is a constant variety of patients who are often acutely ill when they arrive. One of her patients was a 22 year old single woman who had tried to commit suicide by taking an overdose of drugs and was brought to the hospital by police officers.

Among the occupational therapy goals established was decreasing the patient's dependency on staff and simultaneously increasing her interaction with her co-patients. Beverly found it was important to have the patient recognize the need to plan for future vocational goals. Beverly worked with the patient on preparation for the high school equivalency examination. It was necessary for Beverly to remind the patient to focus on her school work. When her medication caused blurred vision, Beverly read to the patient and helped her to study. Beverly realized that it was important to be both honest and clear to help the patient to know that she was expected to focus on the task. Beverly also had to remind herself not to take the patient's mood changes personally.

Since the COTA has to serve as a therapeutic role model, Beverly experienced many feelings which she had to control including frustration and disappointment. But she also enjoyed feelings of accomplishment as she enabled her patient to achieve goals.

Joe works in an *open unit* where patients have privileges to go outside the immediate building and walk around the grounds. One of his patients was a middle-aged woman with poor concentration and attention span. Joe set a specific goal for this patient "the patient will stay with a project for 15 minutes daily, 5 times per week," yet chose a project to meet her individual background. The patient was to paint glaze on a ceramic clay owl which she had chosen to give to one of the doctors. In order to have the patient stay with this project, the COTA permitted her to take a 15 minute cigarette break after each coat of glaze was completed. She was also told that if she stayed with this project until it was finished, she could have a second cup of coffee. This activity went quite well, but further work was needed to promote involvement and neatness.

Another activity for the patient was designed to increase her self esteem and interaction with others. Noticing that the patient handled make-up well, the COTA was able to structure a situation in which the patient helped other patients apply make-up. She accepted cigarettes and coffee in exchange for her expertise. This required her to interact with others and at the same time provided recognition for her abilities.

A similar approach was used for a 25 year old, admitted because of bizarre behavior. Joe identified specific problems which he could help the patient to modify. The COTA stated the behavior to be corrected as "The patient does not use his leisure time appropriately in the cafeteria." A specific goal was then identified to meet the problem, "The patient will visit the cafeteria, buy his food, and will not beg others for their foods or cigarettes." Finally, with the help of the OTR supervisor, the COTA decided on the method he would use to achieve the goal. "The patient and I will discuss the appropriate behavior for a person visiting the cafeteria. We will discuss why it's inappropriate to ask other people for their food or cigarettes. The patient and I will then visit the cafeteria and buy snacks, sit and talk and he will demonstrate that he is able to behave appropriately in the cafeteria without reminders."

Ilene, who entered an occupational therapy assistant educational program just after high school graduation, is assigned to the *Intensive Rehabilitation* Building, and finds her work there very satisfying since she has a lot of independence and can see the results of her efforts. Her OTR supervisor is located in another building. Most of Ilene's patients were only receiving custodial care before the rehabilitation unit was created. Ilene and other young staff were hired to provide an energetic approach to the challenge of introducing active therapy for patients who had been institutionalized for years.

Through a grooming program Ilene was able to get patients who had hardly looked at a mirror in years to recognize themselves and begin everyday practices such as brushing teeth and combing hair.

As a COTA, Ilene is responsible for an ongoing in-hospital shopping program as well. She uses a room as a store and keeps it well stocked with ready-to-eat items and essentials. She encourages patients to participate in making decisions and handling responsibilities by distributing money and vouchers to them and letting them know that they will be able to buy refreshments at the store. Those who attend the morning community meeting where staff and patients have an opportunity to share information, receive the store vouchers. The COTA supervises which patients may go to the store and how many are on line at the store window at any given time. At all times, one staff member and one patient work in the store.

Ilene uses positive reinforcement with the patients in her unit in other activities including keeping their beds and belongings neat as preparation for possible discharge to a community setting. Ilene also selects those patients who may be ready to handle actual paid work tasks. She then assigns them to a work task group on the unit. If their work skills prove to be adequate, she then refers them to the hospital's vocational training program.

Partial Hospitalization Program

David immigrated to the U.S. with his family and entered occupational therapy assistant school after completing a High School Equivalency program. David works in a partial hospitalization program in life skills training. The other staff members in his department include community liaison workers, activity therapists, art therapists and occupational therapists. A partial hospitalization program might refer to a half-way house where a participant spends either the day or night in the psychiatric facility. Remaining time is spent in the community. Figure 9-1 shows preparation for an evening program for those who return to the hospital after work or school during the day.

One of David's patients, a 32 year old man who had led a sheltered life with his grandparents, was seen by David four times a week. Since his grandparents' death, the patient was depressed and unable to do any of the day-to-day things required to care for himself alone.

To help the patient see himself in a realistic manner, David worked with him in a role playing group two times a week. This group allowed the patient to socialize with others and to give and receive feedback.

To increase his self-esteem, the patient was assigned a leather kit project which he could complete easily. To increase the client's work tolerance, David considered both the client's interest as well as the need for a long-term project and chose to have him make a wooden napkin holder. Although he initially resisted the task, with repetition the patient was able to complete it. As a result he was referred for vocational training toward marketable skills.

Single Room Occupancy Housing Program/Shelter for Homeless

Mary serves as a COTA in what is called a single room occupancy (SRO) building, essentially an apartment house where persons receiving social service or welfare benefits may be housed inexpensively. Many former patients, discharged from state psychiatric centers, are found in single room occupancy buildings or shelters for the homeless. Therefore, outreach programs may be provided for them in order to prevent reinstitutionalization. (These are sometimes newly identified with "street psychiatry" for the homeless.) As part of a team Mary visits the building three times each week hoping to facilitate clients' adjustment to the community. She leads activity groups, encourages self care and socialization, takes residents to existing community programs, and tries to get family or visitors involved in productive interaction and activity with the residents.

Chemical Dependency Unit (Substance Abuse Program)

Chris is an occupational therapy assistant in a chemical dependency unit for alcoholics and drug abusers. Her patients are generally educated and hold middle class jobs. One of the goals of occupational therapy in this setting is to help bolster self-confidence among recovering patients, as a low self-image may have contributed to drug or alcohol abuse in the first place. Chris's supervisor believes that occupational therapy offers patients the "high" they got from drugs through activities they enjoy and are good for them. Chris, whose responsibilities include preparing materials for a group, generally allows patients to pick activities in which they are interested, although she might, for example, steer a person with a short attention span towards an activity that would help his concentration. The learning and crafts lab includes equipment for basic wood and leatherwork, needlecraft, ceramics (as shown in Figure 9-2) and basketry. Chris enjoys the opportunity to assist in a program which is designed to change an alcohol and drug dependent lifestyle to one which is productive and non-addictive.

IN THE WORDS OF AN OCCUPATIONAL THERAPY ASSISTANT

After approximately 18 years of involvement with the physically handicapped, I was offered an opportunity to move into the field of psychiatry. The change has broadened my horizons within the profession and has given me new enthusiasm for maintaining my professional position as a COTA within a facility.

Being the COTA on a homemaking rehabilitation training program for the mentally handicapped has provided a challenge to my experience and competence since it required a greater expansion of general knowledge and responsibility vital to the delivery of services within the profession. The responsibility of this program increased my perspective, enhanced my skills, and broadened my learning toward improved care and treatment for the mentally handicapped.

I work alone conducting a vocationally oriented homemaking rehabilitation program designed purposefully and therapeutically to provide patients with an informal home like atmosphere while training them to re-enter community life.

This program is located in a two-story structure off the immediate hospital grounds. My position is to provide learning experiences for patients via meal planning, preparation, nutritional values, (as shown in Figure 9-3) housekeeping, grocery shopping, community trips, money management, self-care, social and communication skills. Visual aids, films, current events, formal/informal dining, family style eating together, and personal development discussions are conducted regularly to encourage further awareness and are important to the education of the individuals. The Home Arts program treats many psychiatric diagnoses. Ages range from 20 through 70. A maximum of 12 to 14 male and female patients are treated daily on a 5-day per week basis with the scheduling of two groups per day. The program is arranged for 10 weeks per patient.

Contact and consultation are held regularly with the unit OTRs. Patients receive initial evaluations by unit OTRs prior to entry to Home Arts. They receive screening and re-evaluations by the COTA during the 10-week program.

This is a good position for the COTA because it allows one to be creative and use the various skills and knowledge acquired via technical training and daily experience. It allows for the COTA to regain and maintain a sense of worth for services. It gives one a feeling of efficiency and effectiveness of self, and allows for the use of judgement and confidence. It encourages the COTA to feel proud of being a COTA, not for monetary purposes, but for the opportunity to expand the program needs and make contact with others.[25]

Beatrice White, COTA
Springfield Hospital Center
Sykesville, MD

IN THE WORDS OF AN OCCUPATIONAL THERAPY ASSISTANT

I enjoyed working with special education adolescents but didn't want a career in teaching. I checked out OT and social work, and OT was more involved with patients, so I chose it as a career. I was very happy to hear all about the wide range of facilities we are able to work with in home health care, hospitals, schools, etc.

I began an OTA program in 1980. The program interested me because I always enjoyed working with the physically impaired and I chose to work at this psychiatric hospital as a mental health worker in the clinical department because I had had no experience with psychiatric patients.

There are two other COTAs employed here, but they work in the activities department.

My job consists of working one to one with patients, developing treatment plans, offering work to deal with anger, organizing and running two activities of daily living and dependent care groups along with goal setting and goal feedback. I also take my adolescents off-grounds once a week, write progress notes in charts, and participate in a school program that we provide in our hospital setting, a 60 bed psychiatric hospital.

I hope at some point to work with the Special Olympics, and become some type of director of the program.

Lindasue Doornbos
Grand Rapids, MI

SUGGESTIONS

1. Contact your local mental health association for general information on mental health.
2. Contact a local occupational therapist or assistant working in mental health to ask whether you may observe or volunteer.
3. Visit a community based mental health program.
4. Examine your feelings about persons with emotional problems.
5. Learn about a crisis intervention hotline number.

READING OBJECTIVES

1. Describe the types of persons served by mental health programs.
2. List ways in which a mental health client may benefit from occupational therapy.
3. Identify courses or subjects that prepare an occupational therapy assistant to work in mental health.
4. Give examples of treatment settings and the type of occupational therapy provided.

REFERENCES

[25]Excerpts from The Homemaking Program for the Mentally Handicapped, Occupational Therapy News, 1984.

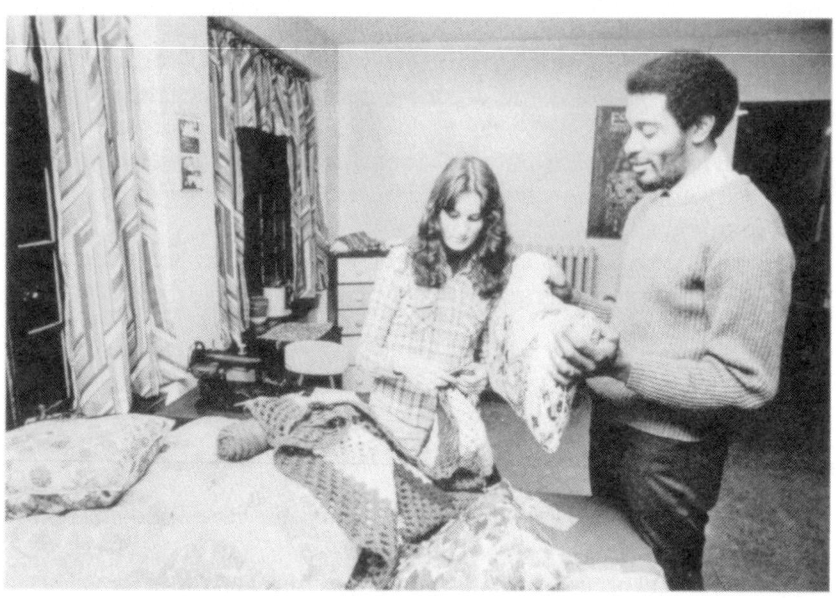

Figure 9-1: With some help from her COTA fieldwork supervisor an occupational therapy assistant student prepares for an evening craft group session at a state psychiatric center "Hotel" program for patients who go out to jobs or school during the day.

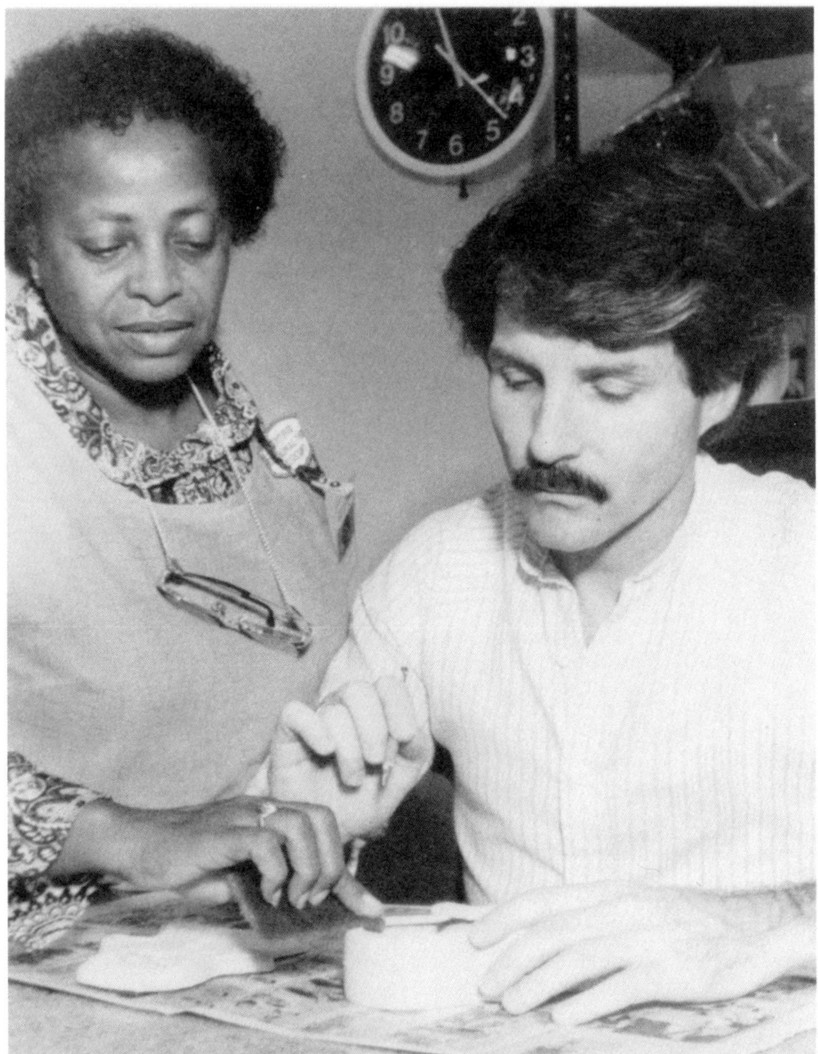

Figure 9-2: Ceramics is one of the important therapeutic activities used in occupational therapy. Physically it provides for fine movements such as pinch, forward and backward motions of the shoulder through rolling, full hand stretching while flattening clay, and grasp for handling tools. In mental health it can be an outlet for hostility when pounding clay to remove air bubbles, an opportunity to experience "messy" items in a socially acceptable way, and a means to achieve self satisfaction through the finished product. Here the COTA demonstrates a technique for smoothing a plaster form after it is taken from a mold. Photo Credit: Elaine H. Jones, "Pop Art Productions" for Creative Business Services, Florida, 1983.

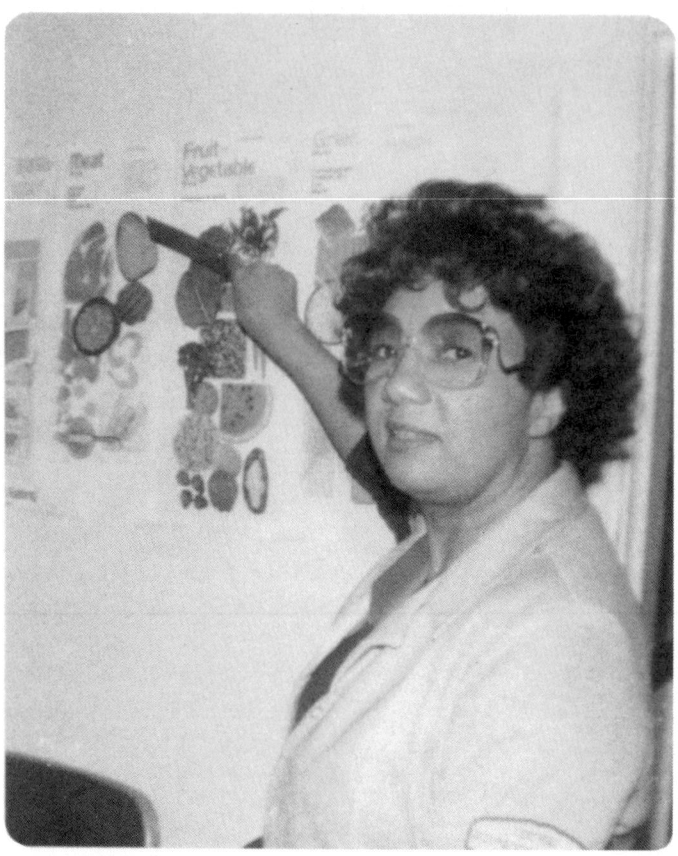

Figure 9-3: A homemaking program involves the COTA in roles which include meal planning and personal development discussions with clients.

CHAPTER 10

THE OCCUPATIONAL THERAPY ASSISTANT WORKS WITH THE PHYSICALLY CHALLENGED

THE OCCUPATIONAL THERAPY ASSISTANT IN PHYSICAL REHABILITATION

What is Meant by Physical Rehabilitation?

The word physical refers to the body. Rehabilitation is the process of restoring to health or efficiency. Thus, persons who had previously been well but suffered injury or illness would be serviced through a physical medicine and rehabilitation program. This might include the permanently disabled or those with a temporary weakness or fracture. Hemiplegia (half sided paralysis resulting from a stroke) is one of the conditions most frequently treated by the occupational therapy assistant. Persons with other chronic diseases including arthritis and multiple sclerosis also benefit from occupational therapy. Persons with illnesses such as heart disease, and cancer or those who have had accidents resulting in limited movement or sensation might also be referred for occupational therapy. Even surgical treatment (such as removal of a breast) might be followed by occupational therapy to restore strength and full range of movement that the person previously had experienced.

At the 1984 International Games for the Disabled (Olympics) the opening address identified the participants as "physically challenged," a positive description.

Where are the Physically Challenged Treated?

General hospitals frequently have a physical medicine and rehabilitation service. Independent rehabilitation centers may admit all those with physical disabilities or may specialize in a particular kind of patient. Skilled nursing facilities (often called nursing homes) provide rehabilitation services for those adults of any age who have conditions that require treatment beyond the time of their hospitalization and also service those with long-term illnesses. In addition to places where the physically disabled receive round the clock services, there are non-residential settings such as out-patient clinics or ambulatory care services or hospital based programs. Rehabilitation centers treat in-patients, out-patients or both. Clients might be seen for day treatment or for specialty services. Occupational therapy is also provided through home care programs and through voluntary agency community based projects as shown in Figure 10-1.

What Does the Occupational Therapy Assistant Need to Know?

In order to properly treat the person with physical impairment, the assistant must first learn basic information about the body and how it works. The student learns about the muscles, bones and nerves of the body and how they coordinate together to create normal movement. Other systems of the body such as the cardiovascular system, are studied as well. Basic science courses include biology or anatomy and physiology. After learning about how the body functions, grows and develops, the student learns about the diseases that affect the normal process and what can be done about them.

Cases, symptoms and treatment are presented for medical conditions which occupational therapy assistants are most likely to encounter.

The student also learns about other members of the rehabilitation team, such as physical therapists and speech therapists, how they are trained and the kind of responsibilities they carry out. Examples are given of how different health professionals work together for the best treatment of the patient. The occupational therapy assistant learns about health care legislation, how departments in a hospital or rehabilitation center are organized and who might supervise and/or refer patients to occupational therapy.

Following this fundamental knowledge, the occupational therapy assistant must learn the specifics of occupational therapy in physical rehabilitation. The assistant will learn special techniques in activities of daily living including how a shirt can be put on using only one arm and hand, or how to use a long handled brush when bending or reaching are not possible. The student will learn to make devices which assist a person to carry out self care, for instance to build up a handle on a spoon or fork so that a person with weak grasp can use it and to assist in assigning tasks and observing the client at work to assess his or her abilities to carry out specific skills required for a job.

The assistant will learn skills and activities that can be used therapeutically including games and crafts that may be structured to require coordination of parts of the body, such as ball playing, checkers or woodworking. In addition knowledge of the use of specified equipment is important.

The OTA may be required to train a patient to use a wheelchair or introduce a task which requires finger manipulation. Newer equipment includes the use of the computer for communication and perceptual skills training.

The assistant must also know the goals of OT in physical rehabilitation and which activities might be used to meet such goals. The student learns principles in the classroom and then has an opportunity to apply them in the clinical setting under direct supervision during required field work.

The occupational therapy assistant student learns about architectural barriers and how the environment may be adapted to meet the needs of a client. Training of the "handicapped homemaker," an important responsibility of the occupational therapy assistant (Figure 10-2) is an example of this. An angled mirror over the stove enables a person in a wheelchair to see inside the pot from a seated position. Front button controls on the stove are easily accessible and require little strength or movement. An adapted cutting board has suction cups to stabilize it and two stainless steel nails to hold a vegetable while it is cut or peeled using one hand.

The student also learns about the importance of dealing with the psychological aspects of physical disability. A movement group is an example of an activity that meets both physical and psychological needs and may be used in a variety of settings. Students are given an opportunity to lead their classmates (Figure 10-3) in such activities and receive feedback from them. A movement group maintains range of motion in the joints, gives a feeling of belonging while not requiring direct interaction, provides an opportunity for following directions, and promotes both physical and mental health.

The occupational therapy assistant student must also learn the uses of a number of items made specifically for therapeutic purposes. These include a type of plastic putty which can be pinched off in bits or stretched for fine and gross movement and a stretchable band (shown in Figure 10-5 being demonstrated by an occupational therapy assistant student) which can be cut to size and comes in different strengths for added resistance.

The different roles and responsibilities of the occupational therapist and occupational therapy assistant are clarified and experienced both in the classroom and in the field.

Opportunities

The specialty of physical rehabilitation has been a continuous area of employment of the OTA. The majority of occupational therapy assistants in the area of physical disabilities work with a varied population and use many different therapeutic approaches. However, occupational therapy assistants have specialized as well. There are OTAs who exclusively make splints, work in burn centers, direct sheltered workshops or other vocational rehabilitation programs, train amputees, instruct handicapped homemakers, service the spinal cord injured, or work in hospitals, nursing homes and rehabilitation centers. However, increasing numbers work in the community, in home care programs and with voluntary agencies such as the Multiple Sclerosis Society. Examples of OTAs in practice in adult physical dysfunction settings follow.

EXAMPLES OF OCCUPATIONAL THERAPY ASSISTANTS WORKING WITH THOSE WITH VARIOUS PHYSICAL CHALLENGES IN A VARIETY OF SETTINGS

Rehabilitation Center—Head Trauma and Epilepsy

Vera, the occupational therapy assistant, was assigned to a 24 year old male who was admitted following hospitalization for a blow to the head. The patient had been living with his parents while attending college as a business management student. After the injury a steel plate was surgically inserted in the patient's head. The patient was left with paresis (weakness) on the right side of the body, difficulty expressing his thoughts verbally and poor perception and learning skills. He was referred for rehabilitation evaluation.

The patient was found to perform more effectively on untimed tasks. Vera worked with him to increase his work speed and self confidence as well as to explore vocational strengths.

The patient was supplied with adaptive devices planned in occupational therapy including a clip-on brace for the right shoe, a shoulder harness to aid in keeping the arm supported in the right position and a hand splint to keep the fingers from curling into the hand.

Skilled Nursing Facility—Below Knee Amputation

Among the occupational therapy assistant's assigned residents was a 71 year old woman whose amputation was surgically performed at a general hospital following an injury. Subsequently she received occupational therapy at a rehabilitation center where she learned to transfer to a wheelchair, chair, bed, and toilet using her prosthesis (artificial leg).

Shiela, the occupational therapy assistant, worked with the patient to increase strength in her upper extremities using a weighted pulley, inclined sander, and arm support aid. The patient lifted a weighted cane above her head and used a five pound bowling ball to hit pins. The occupational therapy assistant provided activities of daily living training for the patient with a walker. She also reviewed safety precautions, trained the patient to brush her hair standing in front of a mirror, covered mouth hygiene standing in front of a sink, and demonstrated dressing and wheelchair mobility. The occupational therapy assistant worked to increase the patient's attention span via making a mosaic ashtray and a hooked rug. Increased socialization was offered through small group activity such as card playing.

Orthopedic Unit of Medical Center—Fractured Hip

Michael, the COTA found that "fractured hip" was the main diagnosis on his orthopedic unit. Through on-the-job training he learned a lot about total joint replacements. He works independently with patients on dressing and bathing skills, provides activities to increase leisure time use and teaches work simplification skills in homemaking.

One patient was a 55 year old former dancer who was hit by a motorcycle. The occupational therapy treatment for this patient included independence in self care, bed mobility and transfers. The COTA began step-by-step working on goals one at a time, for example: strengthening arms which would be needed to push up from a chair, then a standing pivot transfer to a chair. The COTA followed guidelines used by his supervisor for an activities daily of living evaluation.

Lifting bean bag weights on a dowel and small dumb-bells and playing ball were used to increase strength and endurance. The patient practiced transferring to different types of chairs—with and without armrests, and to toilet and bed. He practiced simple kitchen activities washing a dish and making coffee. There were precautions during exercise and sitting. Certain motions, including hip flexion, adduction and internal rotation, were avoided.

The patient had difficulty remembering instructions and safety precautions and needed close supervision, and the occupational therapy assistant had to provide a lot of encouragement and sometimes physical assistance.

This patient, if not treated by occupational therapy, would have remained dependent in all self care skills. The patient didn't engage in any social interaction with other patients in the room unless the COTA arranged it. The COTA assisted with making foot splints which definitely helped relieve the patient's skin ulcers. A re-motivation group and group craft activity helped relieve the patient's boredom with treatment and his general disinterest in his environment.

Independent Living Center—Multiple Sclerosis with Visual Changes

The occupational therapy assistant, Bertha, primarily sees clients in their own homes. She uses the independent living center for office space and to plan supplies and materials for home visits.

One of her medical patients has multiple sclerosis. He experienced gradual changes with the first indication of incoordination, grogginess and a flat facial expression. Within two to three years he developed blurred and double vision. The progression twenty years later included difficulties with vision and speech and tremor when trying to use his hands. Later the patient developed weakness in his legs. He was hospitalized with left hemiparesis, reversed cervical spine curvature, and 80% spinal cerebellar degeneration. He now also has arteriosclerotic heart disease and hypertension. The patient was prone to falls in which he had sustained several fractures. At one time he had been a heavy drinker but had replaced drinking with gambling. The patient was 54 years old, and lived alone. Although the patient wasn't wheelchair bound he had limited mobility which added to his frustration. A home health aide did his cooking, laundry, and shopping. Bertha discussed with the patient approaches toward safety of his bathroom including installing grab bars in the tub and near the toilet. The patient's appearance was neat and clean. He had concern and the willingness to do as much as possible for himself. When he could no longer manipulate buttoning shirts, velcro closures were advised and provided to enable him to continue caring for himself.

Bertha worked with the patient twice a week for movement exercise to improve coordination and increase muscle strength. She encouraged him to rest between exercises.

Chronic Disease Hospital—Spinal Cord Injury

Priscilla, the occupational therapy assistant, works with a variety of patients who have had spinal cord injuries. Many are young men who have been paralyzed from the neck or waist down.

The occupational therapy plan is to increase muscle strength, endurance, self-care skills, and sitting balance. Priscilla worked with one patient twice daily in the clinic, twice at bedside, and once in Ceramics Group. Each session lasted one hour. In the clinic she utilized active range of motion exercises, graded resistive exercises, trunk rotation exercise, and provided a lot of psychological support. She assisted in an occupational therapy and physical therapy evaluation of the patient for use of a sliding board to transfer from wheelchair to bed. At bedside the patient was able to bathe and groom except for her back. Priscilla gave her a long handled sponge and instructed her to use it to clean her back.

Ceramics Group provided an opportunity for the patient to see she was still capable of engaging in productive activity and to have a chance to talk with other spinal cord injured persons.

General Hospital—Heart Disease

Irene works in a program for heart disease patients. One of Irene's patients had been a social worker for a good many years until she retired at 66. She had arteriosclerotic cardiovascular disease and congestive heart failure. The change of life-style was very upsetting to her and she became depressed. Irene worked with the patient to overcome her depression and found different avenues to occupy her time.

Irene's treatment plan developed with the OTR consisted of the following goals: increasing active range of motion and muscle power in both arms, increasing grasp strength in both hands and providing projects of interest for the patient to increase her self esteem. The modalities used were a weighted baton, a finger climbing board, Theraplast (like stretchable clay) and a mosaic tile project.

Home Care—Stroke

Amy carries out her occupational therapy assistant responsibilities in the individual homes of her patients or clients. Her primary case load consists of patients living in the community who have been referred for occupational therapy by Visiting Nurse Service, home health agencies or by private physicians. After the occupational therapist evaluates the patient Amy is assigned to implement part of the treatment plan.

One of her patients was a veteran who had worked as a farmer and mechanic before a stroke (cerebral vascular accident) which left him with a half-sided paralysis. Amy demonstrated dressing techniques such as putting his paralyzed arm into a shirt first while placing it on his lap. She also showed him how to prepare meals while his wife was out working, by using devices such as a cutting board with stainless steel nails to hold a potato so that it could be peeled with one hand. She set up a communication board so that he could make his needs known by pointing to the word or object since his speech was no longer understandable. She played checkers and a bean bag toss game with him to improve his cognition and perception and his upper extremity function while at the same time giving him a sense of achievement.

Amy will sometimes make a home visit with or for a hospitalized patient who is expected to be discharged back in the community. This might involve checking out the width of doorways or the height of cabinets to assess whether the patient could manage in a wheelchair. Amy deals with both the physical and psychological needs of her clients in the home. She helps them develop leisure activities to productively occupy their many hours alone. She trains them in self care activities within their limitations and provides for special devices where indicated. Also, she carries out therapeutic exercise programs for increasing strength or range of motion within the treatment plan written by the OTR.

Amy must be sensitive to the particular environment of the home including the physical facilities (as shown in Figure 10-2) as well as the family members. She uses the trunk of her car as a mobile office. It contains a file drawer with resource materials, boxes of craft materials, equipment that is small enough to be easily transported, assistive devices for self care, and small items for therapeutic exercise and perception training.

Since she is usually on her own, Amy must be sure she has brought all the necessary items with her, has checked with the OTR in advance regarding any questions, and observes all safety precautions. She likes the feeling of independence she has in home-care and the variety of working in a different location each day. Some patients are seen only once for a special need while others are seen once or twice each week.

Pain Management Clinic—Arthritis

Alice was hired as an occupational therapy assistant shortly after the clinic opened when it was recognized that the skills of an occupational therapy assistant in this program would be valuable. She works with clients who range in age from the upper teens through the 90s. The clients have pain which may have originally been related to an orthopedic condition but which lingers and cannot be relieved through usual treatment procedures.

Alice finds her role quite diversified and respected. Her clients include those who have had joint replacements, older individuals with multiple joint pains, an adolescent with limited range of motion in the knee, those who have had back surgery and persons with systemic diseases such as lupus and rheumatoid arthritis.

One such patient was a 45 year old woman who had had rheumatoid arthritis for several years and had tried several treatment approaches. Alice had to work with her on a number of levels. There were family concerns related to her ability to handle various household and self care tasks. Alice invited the family in to observe the client's program and talk about how some of the issues might be resolved. Alice had to deal with both the emotional and physical aspects of the case. The client was depressed and experiencing effects of overuse of medications in her efforts to control pain. Alice included the patient in a craft group which helped her to gain a better self image, to interact with others and to have a new area of focus. The movement group (a type of which is demonstrated in Figure 10-3) which Alice co-led with the occupational therapist and physical therapist also provided a way to meet therapeutic goals directed toward her psychological functioning while at the same time meeting the need to maintain physical range of motion in her joints.

Activities of daily living was another important area which Alice pursued with the patient. Alice showed her ways to dress herself without putting additional stress on the joints, thus reducing pain. Alice also showed her ways to conserve energy in her household tasks such as sliding a filled pot rather than lifting it which again would change the reaction on her arthritic joints. In a short period of time the client made considerable progress managing pain. She was able to increase her functional independence, deal with her family needs better, and recognize her own potential. Alice recalled the client's initial resistance and how several activities had to be tried until one was acceptable. Alice did not want to allow crocheting because of the stress on the finger joints while holding them tightly in one position and wanted an activity that the group could participate in together. She also recalled that the splint that she had helped to make to rest the client's joints at night had brought her concerns and discomfort but was now worn regularly and accepted as providing relief.

Although not all of her cases have a successful outcome, Alice likes the opportunity to try, the short-term nature of the patient contact (usually 3 weeks), and the variety both within her responsibilities and in the type of clients she works with. She participates in work evaluations for workmen's compensation cases, for example giving the client an activity to do while standing and observing the ability to bend over or reach while in that position or the tolerance to standing at a standing table.

IN THE WORDS OF OCCUPATIONAL THERAPY ASSISTANTS

I found myself in two very different settings in my COTA role. The bulk of my experience was in physical rehabilitation centers. One of the centers was in a large mid-western city, part of a complex of medical centers. It was a non-profit, private rehabilitation center. The second center was a rehabilitation setting in a large county hospital in northern California. The expectations for COTAs were significantly different.

While both settings provided continuing education and lectures by visiting therapists and doctors, the private rehabilitation setting provided a more dynamic milieu for a COTA who had expectations for self growth, i.e., learning and taking increased responsibility. In the county rehabilitation setting my responsibility was limited to functional ADL (no crafts). The private rehabilitation center provided the opportunity for teaching and training other COTAs, co-lecturing to OTR interns, making house-visits for assessing discharged patients needs, writing notes to the Visiting Nurse Association, and writing progress and discharge notes (supervised by our OTRs).

I was a liaison between OT and the nursing floor to which I was assigned. I kept nurses and other personnel informed on what OT was doing with individual patients. I also attended medical conferences on my patients.
Marge Harburg, COTA
San Francisco, CA

I decided I wanted to become a COTA after a member of my family had occupational therapy when she was in the hospital.

I had worked in nursing homes the first two years out of school as a COTA and learned quite a bit about fractured hips, the main diagnosis on the orthopedic unit, especially for total joint replacements. The nursing staff and orthopedic doctors were really beneficial in helping me learn more about orthopedics in general.

The supervision I got was rather informal. I see my supervisor daily, and if I have any problems or questions about a patient, we sit down and talk about it or go see the patient. I'm pretty well on my own. If I do run into problems, I contact the supervisor. I will usually check with her on things such as range of motion and hand functioning exercises. I also give in-service classes to the nursing staff and students.

My day consists of screening patients to see if occupational therapy could be beneficial for them. If so, I will get a referral from the attending doctor for whatever treatment I feel they may need. I try to see patients in the morning for ADL skills and then in the afternoon I will try to see patients for leisure time use.

I am pretty well satisfied with the position that I hold now. I have given thought to becoming an OTR, but I really don't feel as if I am ready to go on to that. I like what I am doing here. My goal now is to enhance the role of occupational therapy in an orthopedic unit, and to have more people (staff and doctors) aware of the importance of occupational therapy in this setting.

Sherri Sims, COTA
Stormont Vail Medical Center
Topeka, Kansas

I became interested in OT as a direct result of being hospitalized at a chronic disease city hospital and receiving OT at that facility. I'm a paraplegic and confined to a wheelchair, but this fact does not limit my performance.

When I began working at the chronic disease hospital as an OT aide, I had some previous expertise in woodworking. My job at that time was making specialized equipment for patients such as boards to fit over the arms of wheelchairs, sliding boards to help patients transfer from bed to wheelchair, and book stands. I was encouraged by staff to go to college and become a COTA so that I could work more directly with patients.

My job duties now include working with patients on a one to one basis in activities such as woodworking. I co-lead an activity group for patients who need to maintain strength and movement in their arms. My favorite group is one that I lead alone, a wheelchair basketball group. I continue to make adapted equipment, but with the new perspective of understanding the theory behind it and with the ability to utilize my own ideas as well as those of the professional OTRs.

I have the ability to empathize and relate to the patients on a social level. I feel that they relate and work well with me.

Charles Gray, OTA
Goldwater Hospital
Roosevelt Island

Independence means different things to different people. In my job, it may mean teaching a quadriplegic who used to be a secretary how to use various pieces of equipment so that she can write again. It might mean helping a wheelchair bound woman manage vegetable gardening by planting tomatoes and green peppers in flower boxes on her deck. It might be as basic as helping someone learn to brush his teeth again or as complicated as finding ways for a paralyzed homemaker to prepare meals again from scratch.

We look at every aspect of patients' lives, at what they want to do, need to do and can do to be as functional as possible. And often they do more than they think they can. It's a gradual process; you don't just walk in and say, "You're going to dress yourself today." Some patients may master washing their face in a day or so; others are scared, so devastated by what's happened to them that they're not sure of their own worth or capabilities. Those patients I take slower, to give them some very simple, basic successes. Step by step, they become a little more motivated to see that, yes, they can do something.

I enjoy what I do, seeing people make gains. The patient and I do it together. All my patients are unique. Each one is a challenge because their capabilities, their personalities and their goals are all different. What keeps me going, even when progress is slow, is seeing people feel worthwhile again, knowing that I'm part of a profession that can have such a profound effect on other people's lives.[26]
Sandy Dodge, COTA
University of Michigan Hospitals
Employee of the Month

SUGGESTIONS

1. Visit a physical rehabilitation program.
2. Compare programs offered on an in-patient and on an out-patient or home care basis.
3. Find out about stroke, arthritis and other chronic conditions treated by occupational therapy assistants.
4. Talk to someone who has had occupational therapy or rehabilitation services following an injury.
5. Consider how your own or a family member's life style might be affected if physically challenged.
6. Think about some approaches to handle daily living tasks more efficiently.
7. Look at "devices" for sale in ordinary stores or catalogues such as kitchen gadgets or long handled shoe horns and reflect on how they may be helpful for a person who is physically challenged.
8. Visit a rehabilitation equipment store or company or send for a catalogue to learn about items such as that shown in Figure 10-2.

9. Write to an association such as the Parkinson's Disease Foundation or Multiple Sclerosis Society for information about the disorder.

READING OBJECTIVES

1. Compare the term "physically challenged" with physically disabled.
2. Give examples of treatment approaches and materials used in occupational therapy with the physically challenged.
3. List types of disabilities and types of treatment settings served by the occupational therapy assistant.

REFERENCES

[26]Excerpts from Dodge helps Disabled Declare Independence. University of Michigan Hospitals Star, August 31, 1984.

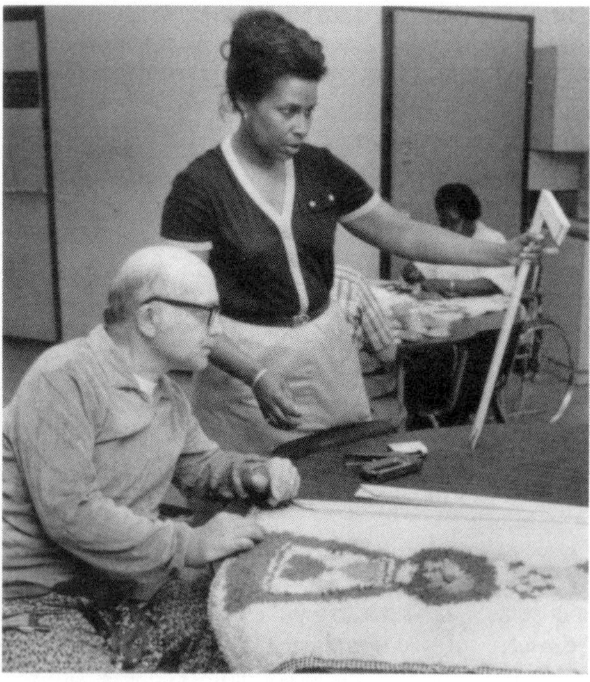

Figure 10-1: Occupational therapy assistant and client making decisions together regarding a frame for the multiple sclerosis patient's just completed hooked rug project which helped to enhance his eye hand coordination and give him a sense of accomplishment.

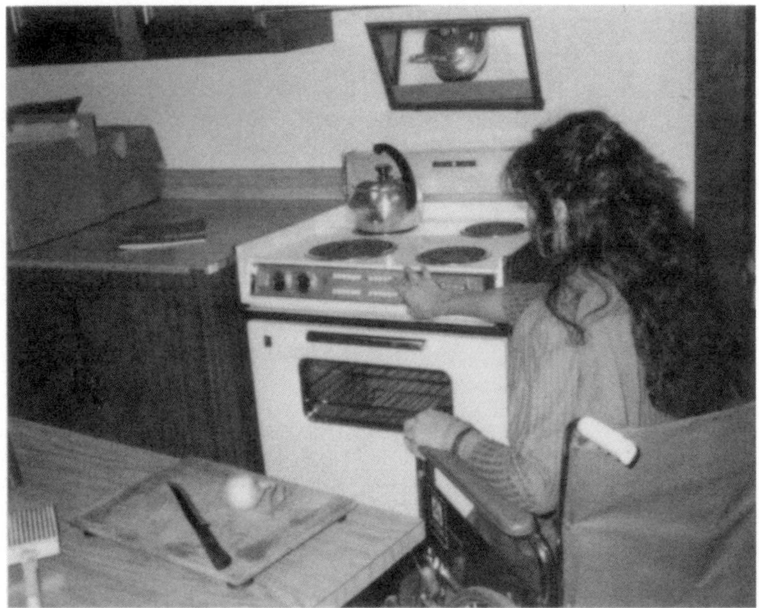

Figure 10-2: Training the handicapped homemaker often involves the use of specially designed or adapted equipment.

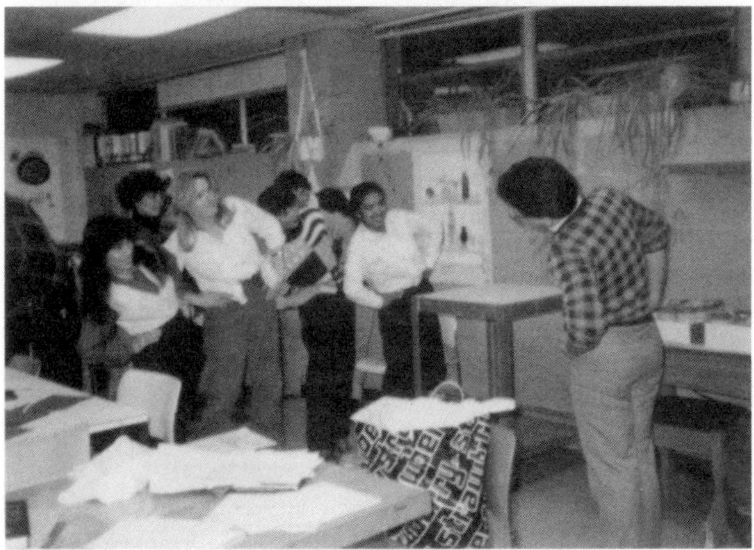

Figure 10-3: Participants in a movement group derive both emotional and physical benefits.

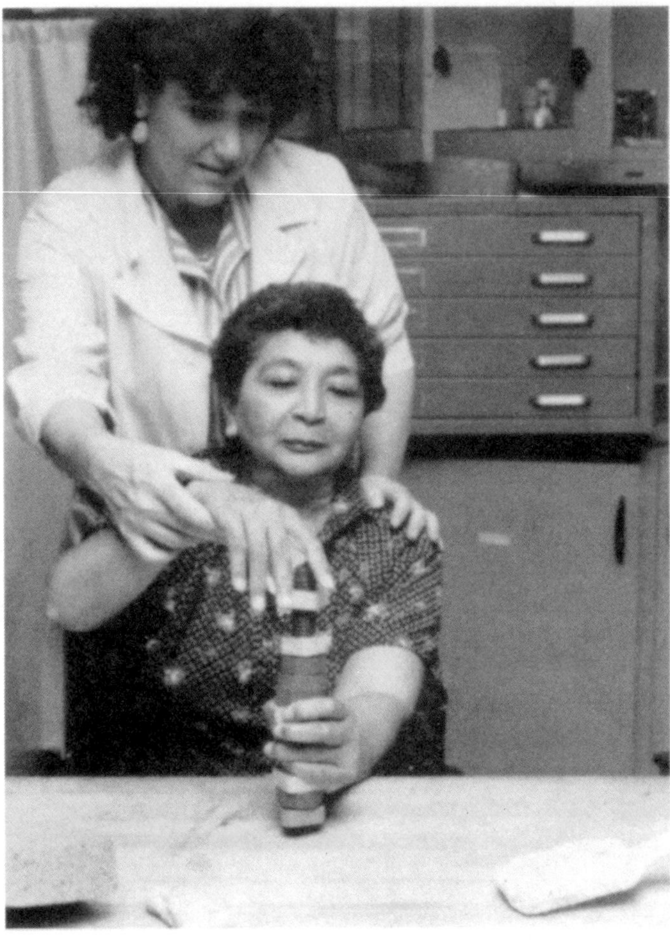

Figure 10-4: An occupational therapy assistant directs proper use of the arthritic wrist for the appropriate therapeutic exercise as her patient carries out the assigned activity.

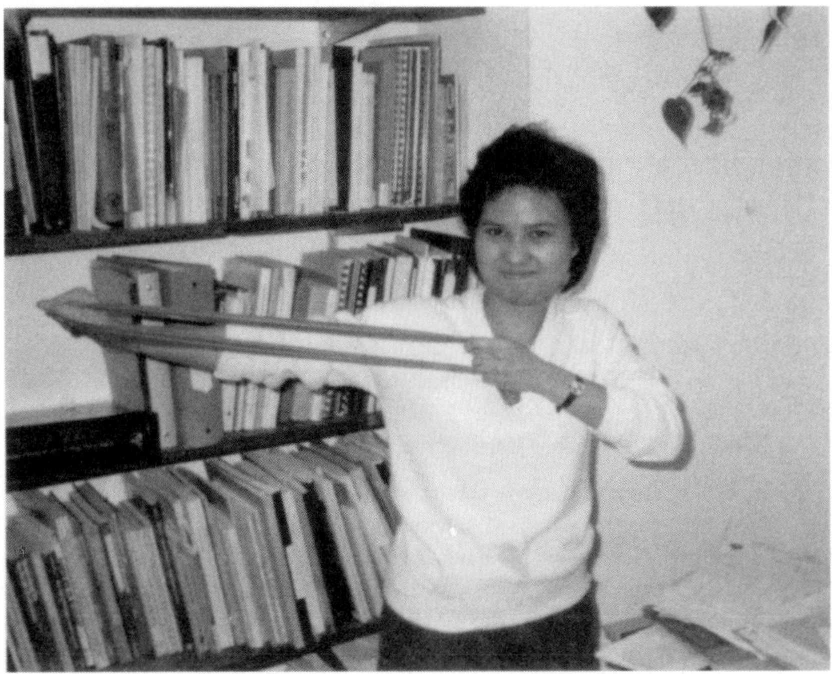

Figure 10-5: An occupational therapy assistant student demonstrates the use of Thera Band for achieving a particular movement.

CHAPTER 11

OCCUPATIONAL THERAPY ASSISTANTS IN EXPANDED ROLES AND SETTINGS

THE OCCUPATIONAL THERAPY ASSISTANT IN EXPANDING ROLES AND SETTINGS

What Kind of Settings are Considered Non-Traditional or Unique?

The occupational therapy assistant traditionally works in five main areas of practice: mental health, physical dysfunction, pediatrics, developmental dysfunction and aging. There are, of course, some areas of overlap as two of the areas above are age designations while the others are identified by dysfunction.

Likewise, many of the non-traditional roles and settings described below may be classified within one of the above categories. However, they have been selected for inclusion in this section as few occupational therapy assistants actually practice in the roles and settings described, though these opportunities are now expanding.

Directors of occupational therapy assistant training programs, identified the following as either non-traditional roles or expanded career opportunities pursued by their OTA program graduates: respite care worker, home trainer, parks department program director, placement services coordinator, private practice clinician, pain clinic therapist, splinting expert, rehabilitation salesperson, hand therapist assistant, teenage accident victim program supervisor, demonstrator of hospital equipment, residential facility houseparent, children's center program director, brace department supervisor, sheltered workshop evaluator, adult day care counselor, community living trainer, junior or community college instructor, rehabilitation videotape producer, professional conferences coordinator, and facilitator for the deaf or deaf blind. Although occupational therapy assistants working in public schools were once considered unique, changing legislation has increased their presence in that setting.

A look at listings in the "Member Hotline" column of the Occupational Therapy Newspaper or in national and state conference programs shows an additional array of areas in which occupational therapy assistants are practicing. These include: stress center, therapeutic horseback riding, adolescent chemical dependency unit, poetry therapy, burn unit, horticultural therapy, college laboratory technician, educational fieldwork coordinator, adaptive equipment specialist, high school pre-vocational classes, correctional facilities and forensic units, kidney dialysis programs, and cancer care and hospice programs.

What Training Prepares the Occupational Therapy Assistant for Unique Roles and Settings?

The variety of non-traditional responsibilities reflects the variety of experiences in an occupational therapy assistant curriculum. The teaching skills that the student develops to use with a patient might be used instead for college instruction; the foundation training in adapted equipment and splinting can be expanded with additional training or experience to special expertise; the knowledge of physical dysfunctions and approaches to achieving independence despite deficits helps in selling rehabilitation equipment; the exposure to leading groups and administering an activity unit is used in coordinating or directing programs; learning to identify and foster achievement of goals in the psychosocial areas and awareness of the psychological aspects of physical disability prepares an occupational therapy assistant to work in such areas as hospice programs for the dying, pain clinics and kidney dialysis units; the concept of "therapeutic use of self" which is fostered in the training of an occupational therapy assistant is particularly relevant in correctional facilities and community living programs; the inclusion within the curriculum of pre-vocational exploration and vocational adjustment experience enables the graduate to apply these approaches in vocational programs in a variety of settings.

Occupational therapy assistants may, of course, use their own special interests or skills to initiate their unique positions or roles or utilize their OTA training in combination with specialized training to achieve a particular goal. Often OTAs with special abilities are recognized in a traditional role and thus asked to take on expanded responsibilities accordingly.

OPPORTUNITIES AND TRENDS

The position of occupational therapy assistant is relatively new. As an increasing number of occupational therapy assistants accumulate experience in traditional settings, they begin to seek and explore new opportunities. Many of the roles listed above could be filled by persons trained in a variety of ways. The occupational therapy assistant brings a rare combination of skills and knowledge which is increasingly recognized as appropriate for expanding areas in health and community services. New technological developments such as kidney dialysis which requires long passive hours, changing legislation as that requiring mainstreaming of those with dysfunctions into general education facilities, and greater social consciousness including recognizing the need for therapeutic programs for chemical dependency and the homeless all create expanding opportunities for the occupational therapy assistant. The increasing enrollment nationwide in community and junior colleges has not only opened additional positions for occupational therapy assistants as faculty but has increased the awareness of the skills that occupational therapy assistants possess for related areas of practice. The additional attention being paid by the business world to the health of employees has also led to occupational therapy assistants being utilized in executive health maintenance programs, substance abuse efforts and workman's compensation rehabilitation and assessment.

The practice examples which follow are in the actual words of the occupational therapy assistants. The positions listed are at the time the material was collected.

Alcoholism Treatment Program

On the unit my OT program begins with a systematized evaluation procedure for a patient consisting of a task and of an activities of daily living self-report form. This is only administered following a written referral by the attending doctor. Patients are evaluated in a group setting or on an individual basis. For me, there is extensive note writing on initial patient evaluation and on-going treatment.

A very gaunt man we shall call Thomas, shabbily dressed, having only a pair of dirty jeans and a torn shirt, entered the unit. After his detoxification period, I observed his level of self care, awareness, and relationship with others. My evaluation indicated this man needed physical assistance as well as moral support in performing daily living activities. I developed a standard form for recording by the nursing staff and myself the patient's ability or lack thereof to care for his basic needs. I worked with him in daily OT groups and in individual sessions using the laundry and dining room facilities and other communal areas. Some of his distant memory cleared but recent recall was still impaired. It became evident that this former research engineer and Japanese translator would not be able to maintain himself after discharge. The on-going OT evaluation was used by the social worker for aftercare placement.

An increasing number of women with problems of alcoholism have signed themselves into the program. When my initial evaluation shows a contradiction with the patient's self report form of her lifestyle before hospitalization, a home visit is called for. In one case, the patient's children had been away at camp a month. The appearance of her apartment was chaotic. With difficulty, we located long overdue bills and clothing that needed laundering. At the hospital we set up a structured daily schedule in the free time allowed by the program. This was to take care of the patient's immediate needs, like paying her bills and laundering her clothes, giving support and assistance when necessary. The occupational therapy recommendations to the team, were that Sarah would require a homemaker's helper initially and hopefully, with constructive help from her outpatient counselors, Sarah could learn to structure her sober time and use it effectively.

About a third of the patients I treat are possible candidates for the out-reach program. After initial evaluation and other factors indicate they are likely referrals for after-care, the patients are scheduled to my OT workshop. Individual and group tasks (performed for the unit) are either suggested by the occupational therapy assistant or selected by the patient. In an informal setting, no more than eight patients work with the therapist on a parallel (working side by side on individual projects) group level. Individual tasks are usually craft or art projects. For example, copper tooling is one of the media used. Requiring no previous experience, this craft can easily be learned and a picture completed in two one hour sessions. The patient is encouraged to display his project in his own room. Group tasks are projects for decorating the mutual living areas, e.g., a mosaic mural, a hooked wall hanging or maintained plants. The patients also work together on clerical projects for the unit. Patients, through planning, working, and completing a task, can experience a sense of satisfaction as achievement with others in a similar situation. My report on the patients is shared with their OT, working closely on their transition needs. The out-reach OT in single room occupancy housing takes it from there. I conduct a group dealing with the concept of time and of the patients' option to accept the responsibility to change their use of time. If they wish to do so, I have patients work on a visual construction of how they used time before entering the program. The visual might denote "work," "fun," "nothing" or otherwise.

I had been asked to be the representative from the In-Patient Alcoholism Treatment Component to work with six others from the hospital's total alcoholism staff in a pilot program. We planned and developed a new program of patient volunteers from currently attending out-patients. Their jobs are escorting patients from in-patient to out-patient units, to pre-discharge interviews for out-patient care, to social service or welfare offices or other necessary appointments on day of discharge and to provide support during a difficult transition period. Dealing with alcoholics can be a frustrating experience and, as in any field, we have had a high staff turnover on the unit.

As one of the original members of the unit, I see the occupational therapy assistant as one who would require not only the skills of our profession but the ability to adapt to a demanding and dynamic field. To be a positive force in the

patient's treatment, the occupational therapy assistant should be able to communicate on a personal level rather than as a detached clinician. This is vital to a significant patient/therapist relationship.
Winifred Leav, COTA
St. Vincents Hospital
Alcoholism Unit

Brace Department

My office responsibilities include: working directly with the staff doctors of Hand Surgery Associates in the design of orthoses (splints) for congenital birth defects, arthritics, amputees, replantations, burns, and traumatic crush injuries primarily of the upper extremity; supervising design of braces constructed by fellow workers in Brace Department, keeping appropriate records and statistics for each patient including design, type of brace applied, name of doctor in charge of patient, and cost of brace; ordering of supplies for Brace Department; instructing each patient in the proper use and care of the brace and skin care; instructing visiting physicians, occupational and physical therapists in a one week training course in upper extremity orthotics using slides, printed literature, and patient observation; and keeping direct contact with nursing staff to insure that patients leaving the hospital post-operatively are scheduled for appropriate brace application appointments on their return visit to the Hand Clinic.

Before my employment with Hand Surgery Associates, the majority of pre-operative mobilization and immobilization of the upper extremities was achieved with plaster or modification of a prefabricated orthosis. When I joined Hand Surgery Associates I introduced the use of thermoplastics for specialized upper extremity orthotic application. I was asked to design and supervise an upper extremity Brace Department. As the staff of the Hand Surgery Associates became more aware of the advantages of custom made orthoses for post-operative increased recovery time of the patient, first one, then another person was employed and trained by myself to cover the increased use of braces for the growing patient load.
Randall L. Schrock, COTA
Hand Surgery Associates
Supervisor Brace Department
Louisville, Kentucky

Deaf-Blind Program

I told the Office of Vocational Rehabilitation (O.V.R.) that I would like to work with deaf-blind and multi-handicapped youths and adults. O.V.R., which funds training for the deaf and disabled, recommended that I learn to be an occupational therapy assistant. Because of my own deafness the OTA program director told me she could not guarantee placement but worked with me toward it. Before entering my current area of practice, I worked with multi-handicapped workers and clients in the Mayor's Office for the Handicapped, directed training of the deaf at a vocational habilitation center, served as an aide at a school for the deaf, and was a home economics teacher's aide and interpreter for the deaf-blind. I completed the occupational therapy assistant program with the help of sign language interpreters.

I now work at The Institute for the Education of the Blind with rubella children from age 4 to 21 years old, sixty percent of whom are deaf-blind. There are 168 students and 200 staff. The basic Simulated Workshop has a program for low functioning students. I work there as a Pre-Vocational Therapy Assistant, evaluating and simulating work activities. The students are initially evaluated on very simple sorting, packing and assembly and tasks which become more complex as the student progresses. I have the same responsibilities at a second Simulated Workshop for high functioning students. The developmental level of these students doesn't require a one-to-one ratio. The cognitive level shows the students functioning at the 4 year old level or above. The student is independent in basic self-care skills and can be oriented with minimal assistance within buildings and can negotiate simple on-campus mobility routes. I have a supervisor of activities of daily living in the low function workshop and another supervisor in the high function workshop. I also teach sign language to the staff and students.

Marie Kowal
Pre-Vocational Therapy Assistant
Institute for the Blind

Group Home

A friend recommended that I look into the field of OT. I quit my job in a factory and worked for a summer as an aide to an OTR. This work inspired me to pursue a career in OT.

When I worked as a summer aide in several nursing homes I saw how OT could prepare and enable people to deal constructively with their disability. One semester I did independent study/volunteer work in a classroom for mentally impaired high school students. I received an education in vocational training and how the educator can work with the OTR. This inspired me towards work with mentally handicapped.

I am now a live-in assistant in a group home where I live and work with six mentally handicapped adults. I work with 2 other assistants who also live in the home, an old, beautiful house in a residential community.

My work is to assist where necessary. I do some practical household and errand activities while people are away in their workshops. When they are home I assist with cooking, personal care and often simply "being with" the handicapped people. This may mean going to the store, writing a letter, watching T.V., playing music on my dulcimer for all to listen, or taking a walk. We anticipate coming events together and live each day according to our interests and energy level.

One day treasured by each handicapped person is his or her "cook day." I assist one of the persons in my household with cook day. I have structured the pre-planned meal according to a certain order. I may remind the person to defrost the meat in the morning. In the evening I assist by preparing ingredients and watch the timing of recipes. We share serving and prayer during the meal.

OT is valued in my work. I am still convinced that it has much to offer because of its creativity. My first "love" experience with OT was that of having relationships with those who needed medical help. OT can be an advocate for disabled people on a committed basis.

I am also interested in providing OT prevention and health care services to disabled and marginal peoples who cannot afford the costs of private-pay insurance.

David Hesselink, COTA
Live-In Assistant
L'Arche Group Home
Mobile, Alabama

Independent Living Center

My employment as a consultant in an independent living center was through a grant program. Initially my role was seen as a trainer in independent living skills, but it has evolved into providing "link-ups" with other agencies and service providers and cutting red tape. I do still provide training, particularly in the areas of budget and money management and in meal planning. The program is designed to provide services for both the mentally and physically handicapped in a variety of living situations.

Molly Hensel, COTA
Training Consultant
Midland, MI

Kidney Dialysis and Hospice Programs

I have been a COTA working in an acute care setting for 3 years. The programs or diagnoses of patients I have contact with are: Hospice, Oncology Rehabilitation, Kidney Dialysis, burns, total hip replacements, CVA, arthritis, hand and wrist fractures or dislocations.

In the kidney dialysis program OT provides avocational and/or recreational activities to increase and/or maintain upper extremity muscle strength and range of motion, provides diversion to prolonged treatments, helps patients maintain self-worth and productivity, and provides socialization. The COTA is responsible for gathering information about the patent's medical, social and work history, psychological adjustment to treatments, and avocational/recreational interests. By helping to stabilize a project, the therapist becomes available for socialization and psychological support.

In the hospice program the COTA helps to assess dying patients' individual needs and helps these patients maintain their interests for as long as possible e.g., a magnifying glass is used to help a patient with visual difficulties maintain interest in current events. Hospice patients are encouraged to set their own goals. The COTA acts as a facilitator to help stimulate old or new interests to help maintain productivity. Patients often choose to complete a gift for each family member before they die. The in-patient hospice unit is often a teaching center before the patients return home to be with their families. The COTA assesses the patient's self-care level and provides adaptive equipment and instruction in energy conservation before the patient is discharged to hospice home care.

Mary Beth Koski, COTA
St. Mary's Hospital
Milwaukee, Wisconsin

Homemaking Program

As a youngster I worked in camps with the mentally retarded and emotionally disturbed. I knew I enjoyed working with people and I enjoyed crafts and doing things. Eventually I went to the career books, looked to find out what kind of combination I could come up with and saw the listing for an occupational therapy assistant.

As a student I was very interested in homemaking, so I was contacted when the OTR resigned from the program I had trained in. It's one person running an entire area, and I do evaluations and re-evaluations. There's no one cosigning my notes or looking over my shoulder. I am in charge of my area. I am the one doing the telling, setting the goals, writing all of the notes, handling the equipment.

My direct supervision comes from the director of the OT Department. I meet with her once a week to go over any problems I'm having with the work or with the staff. If I need help, I'll talk to the individual therapist working with the patient. I do the planning, maintain the area and do the shopping, keeping the shelves stocked with whatever is needed. I train family members and go over with them what I've been doing with the patient. Once every 3 months I lecture at a stroke family group primarily dealing with one handed techniques. I demonstrate the equipment used with patients and why we use it incorporating cooking, cleaning, shopping and laundry, and concentrating on safety. I meet with clinic representatives once a week to get referrals and to report back on what I'm doing with the patients. I go to rounds twice a week. I think I've seen almost every disease.

As an example, when a paraplegic in a wheelchair is referred to me, I'll ask what the home situation is like and what the needs are in terms of homemaking. Usually it involves a checkout at a standard kitchen height, using the stovetop and the oven safely. I review three basic pieces of equipment with the patient: a mirror that goes over the stove, a low lapboard and a reacher. I will work with the patient and go through a meal, usually a simple meal like breakfast, do the preparation and review some safety precautions.

One of my in-patients is 23 years old and has cerebral palsy. He came in terrified of working in a kitchen area because he was sure he was going to totally mess up and do something very dangerous. The beginning goals were really basic training in a kitchen. His main problem was incoordination; he walked with two crutches. We worked with things like using a rolling cart to transport items back and forth, sitting in a high kitchen chair at a standard height kitchen, and working with very basic recipes. We worked on things like making a bed and vacuuming. We've been concentrating on shopping, because that's been his biggest problem. I see him three times a week for an hour each time. I had him plan a menu of what he wanted to prepare for himself for three days. Menu planning helps energy conservation and cuts down on some of the confusion. From the menu we made a shopping list of items he would need. Then we went to the supermarket to work on things—a problem for him was pushing the cart. He was able to just hold onto one crutch and use the bar of the shopping cart as his additional support. He was terrified and really "bombed out" the first couple of times that we did it. In making the shopping list I helped him to organize it according to dairy products and canned goods. When we got to the supermarket, we reviewed things like getting familiar with where things are, reading the signs in the aisles and then looking at the list, pushing the cart and getting things off the shelves, and checkout. Money management was not a severe problem for him. Scanning was hard. He has some visual problems. He would tend to stand right on top of the area and only see what's right in front of him. So we worked on things like standing back and scanning the shelves to find an item. He's done better, and he's at a point now where in two weeks he'll be discharged from the program and will start looking into housing.

In OTA school the skills courses gave me the basics to work with. My work experience has increased my knowledge. I've looked things up in some of the OT manuals. There are films available that also gave me some additional information and I've learned a lot from the patients. They're the ones doing it. I tell them, "if it's a struggle, let me know that. If you find a way that's easier let me know."

I do go out on home visits, which is an added responsibility that I took on out of my own interest. I've gotten very involved in educating the public. People come in to meet with me who work with the disabled or are disabled themselves and need information. I do work with the families too. I work closely with the vocational counselors, who many times deal with the funding that's needed to get equipment. I worked with a disabled child whose school wanted to know what she was doing in homemaking so that she could get credit for her high school home economics course that she was missing. Being in OT we're exposed to so many different areas and modalities. I'm planning ultimately to work in a training program for community living, using my occupational therapy background.

I'm fortunate that I was given this opportunity. It's a rare position for a COTA to be in. I feel I worked for it. I've done a good job, and I've learned a lot.

Paula Silverman Pendegar, COTA
Homemaking Unit Coordinator
Rusk Institute for Rehabilitation Medicine

Follow up: When I moved to Florida I started out at the bottom. They were unfamiliar with OT and COTAs. I worked my way up to supervisor of a sheltered workshop, then to job placement counselor and eventually to Executive Director of a non-profit organization.

Private Practice

Your first inclination might be to believe that COTA and private practice are incongruous—not so! I think it is becoming increasingly common for COTAs to move beyond the self-imposed limitation of traditional roles and into the realm of innovative, career-oriented practice for professional growth and expansion. COTA practice is only limited by an individual's unwillingness to set a goal and move toward it. Even though COTAs must maintain integrity of practice by functioning within guidelines prescribed by licensure laws and standards for practice, the possibilities remain endless.

When you enter the realm of private practice, another dimension must be considered—beyond the role of occupational therapist, certified. Practicing occupational therapy is the easy part. Numerous years of experience allow movement beyond traditional roles. The dimension to be considered is the business orientation of private practice. Having progressed from experiential learning to formalized education in a Masters Degree program in Business Administration, the supplemental knowledge is invaluable and quite divergent from a human services perspective.

The point to be made is this: formulate a long-range plan (uninhibited by traditional influences); set up short-term objectives along the path to achievement of this goal; pursue the supplemental knowledge/education necessary to

allow for personal and professional growth; and promote a competent self-image as a certified occupational therapy assistant in any chosen area of practice.
Marie A. Rabin, COTA
Partner, Occupational Therapy
Associates Services

Rehabilitation Equipment Company

I am employed by the Home Health Care Department of White and White Inc. as their Rehabilitation Equipment Consultant.

Much of my time is spent in the store helping customers buy or rent durable medical equipment. I am responsible for the ordering and inventory of several of the lines that we carry.

If someone has a question or problem with health care equipment, I am the person they can contact. If I cannot personally help them, I try to refer them to someone on our staff who can.

I am the White & White goodwill ambassador. We are often asked to display our self-help items or called on to explain our services. It is my responsibility to represent our company on these occasions. I have had displays at OT and PT conferences, as well as at Easter Seals Programs, and Indian Trails Handicapped Camp. I have also spoken to nurses aide classes, and to our local OTA program about my job and the services my company offers. I also visit the hospitals and other places that we service to check that their needs are being met.

When someone cannot come to the store, I go to the home to assess their needs. I have measured homebound and nursing home patients for wheelchairs and other equipment. I have done home checks to be sure that the equipment we sell is viable in the home setting. I have also been called upon by OTs and PTs to help pick the correct equipment for a particular patient's needs.

I am proud to be a certified occupational therapy assistant, and I am proud to be an employee of White & White.
Janice Uzarski, COTA
Consultant
Grand Rapids, Michigan

Socialization Program in the Community

I wanted to have a secure profession which paid a good salary. I wanted to work with people, helping. OT offered me games and crafts, something that I had always had a little undeveloped interest in. It offered physical dysfunction as well as psychosocial dysfunction. The areas it could be used in were many. I believe these are some of the things that led me to become a COTA.

This program was started after deinstitutionalization of patients from State psychiatric facilities. The clients range in age from 40 years through the elderly. Their diagnoses are primarily psychiatric, but many have physical problems related to the aging process such as strokes, or have birth defects or mental retardation. The main focus of the program is resocialization, helping the clients cope with their environment, gain appropriate behaviors and deal with the effects of sensory deprivation.

My day starts with a meeting and rounds discussing clients. Afterwards I leave the community center and travel to make contacts with my clients. I usually either engage a client in a craft or game or just talk and encourage social skills. I intervene in problem situations that the client is having and act as advocate for the client in terms of trying to get the needs of the client met. Also, I write in charts each day and I attend team meetings twice a week. I also order supplies. I sometimes attend an inservice training session as well.

Let me describe one case, Mr. H., who had cerebral palsy and has severe contractures of both upper and lower extremities. His speech is slurred and he is mentally retarded. I use various techniques. Maybe I'll use something from a background of sensory stimulation or reality orientation. I also arranged for a pair of properly adapted shoes so that he could participate in activities.

I may use blocks to try to get Mr. H. to improve his coordination. I am also responsible for engaging Mr. H. in some type of social activities, so usually on Thursdays I bring Mr. H. to a group bingo game where I help him put the chips down on his card or just in general socializing with Mr. H.

Another of my cases is Mrs. E. who has relatively high function, is wheelchair bound, and is mildly mentally retarded. In her case I engage her in crafts. Sometimes we use the session to sublimate anxieties that she's having in terms of interactions with other residents or interpersonal problems with the staff. I intervene. I suggest different things to her in terms of activities of daily living and show her different methods that can be used.

Joel Marks
St. Vincent's
Community Outreach Program

Stress Management

As a COTA in a community mental health setting, I function as coordinator of a day treatment care program and stress management program. I'm responsible for planning, budgeting, evaluating and supervision of staff for day and night including screenings, assessments, scheduling, planning and evaluation. For the general activity program I'm responsible for development and planning, inservice training, supervision of staff and of volunteers.

My additional responsibilities include supervision of occupational therapy, human service and social service students, clinical teaching for OT students, ordering supplies, maintaining inventory, program evaluation research, soliciting of donations, and community speaking. I serve as client/patient advocate, liaison with community agencies, custodian for petty cash funds for the mental health auxiliary for outreach programming, liaison with family or family surrogate, and resource consultant for outside agencies. I make home visits, provide crisis intervention, conduct client/staff meetings, interview, assign and schedule volunteers, schedule community speakers or groups for special programs, write monthly reports, conduct inservice training for multidisciplinary staff and handle documentation.

Every day is different from the one before. We service a variety of populations and have a different treatment program each day. Individual sessions are held in the mornings and group sessions in the afternoons. I also work on a stress management program which serves a population that has never been hospitalized or those people who have some degree of abstract thinking and can deal with problem solving and learning stress reduction techniques. Clients in this particular program are part-time or full-time in college or employment. The program is to prevent illness and the need for hospitalization. In the stress program clients have functioned in the community at least marginally, but are more often average or above average in personal, social and occupational roles until numerous stresses precipitate a dysfunction in their ability to adapt to their changing environment. This stress may cause interference with perceptual processing including the possibility of hallucinations. Formerly competent to perform in many roles they are now stressed by simple problem solving or accomplishing of a basic skill to such a degree that they withdraw physically and socially and express great fatigue. I work with them on coping techniques.

I developed a stress history tool in conjunction with the stress reduction program. It helps to identify what methods of stress management have worked or not worked for the individual in the past. Management of stressful problems may include pleasurable exercise, muscle relaxation, guided imagery, sensory words and stimulation, leisure time activities, acceptance of feelings and friendly socialization, and mind bender exercises such as computer games.

I started work as a psychiatric attendant in a mental institution, and at that point in time I did not know that occupational therapy existed. After working for two to three years in an institution with much frustration and not much mobility I began to investigate other job opportunities and am still taking courses. This is an ongoing process. It is something that one must always be mindful of. One needs to keep abreast of current trends and concepts. Before becoming a COTA I had done other craft types of volunteer work with boy scouts and senior citizens. Throughout my OT career I've been involved with professional activities. If one

can demonstrate ability and responsibility, the reward is that you get additional tasks and added responsibility.
Terry Brittell, COTA, ROH
Coordinator Day Treatment
Stress Management Coordinator for staff and patients
Mohawk Valley Psychiatric Center

Outside the USA

The medical center houses two hundred beds, 98 percent occupied. The OT department consists of two OTRs, and 3 COTAs. One OTR works with physical dysfunction patients, perhaps three or four at any given week. The other works with psychiatric patients with the help of a COTA. The third COTA services the therapeutic work program.

The Air Force traditionally allows COTAs to participate and facilitate treatment without direct supervision of an OTR. I run the alcohol rehabilitation portion of the program. I usually have 12–15 patients at a time. The program is a 28 day program with 10 hours of OT clinic a week. Traditional crafts are used to evaluate work and social and cognitive skills, to promote leisure activity skills, self awareness activities and a goals group. I participate in group therapy, recreational therapy, "Big Book" and "Step Study" groups as well as other groups on the ward.
Sgt. Cynthia L. Gomez, COTA
United States Air Force
Regional Medical Center

Occupational Therapy Assistant Curriculum (Figure 11-1)

Initially, I was interested in teaching and completed one year of college. I had a friend enrolled in an OTA program so I visited the school and class and became interested because it was a people oriented profession and had teaching aspects.

I found occupational therapy interesting and very diversified...a job where one could be creative and that wouldn't become rote or boring.

As instructor in a nontraditional occupational therapy assistant program where much of the curriculum is individualized, I write and organize instruction packets (manuals), lecture, demonstrate, correct students' work and supervise 3 week affiliations and field trips. My instruction areas are Psychosocial Function, Assertiveness Training, Basic Grammar and Letter Writing, Therapeutic Aspects of Groups, Media, Social Skills and Theory, Introduction to Holistic Health, Organization and Administration, and Introduction to Geriatrics.

Each job area offers new opportunities and "growth" experiences, so it is

interesting. To be a good COTA one must be assertive and outgoing, have an optimistic outlook on life in general, feel comfortable or willing to try new things, be flexible and always take the initiative to learn more.
Paula Leimer, COTA
Instructor in OTA Program
Duluth Area Vocational Technical Institute
Duluth, Minnesota

Supportive Services and Respite Care

The atmosphere of love and caring fills this lovely home. Mr. B. is a 72 year old man who has aphasia as a result of two CVAs; he has some weakness and lack of fine motor coordination in his right hand. He is a paraplegic due to a clot in the spinal column which occurred at the time of his second stroke. He wears a catheter. After being in a nursing home for 11 months, he returned to his home. During the two-hour morning sessions that I am with Mr. B., we work on bathing, dressing and transfers. While he was in the nursing home he refused to participate in any activities. But for some reason he is willing to do some craft projects with me. He has sanded, stained and varnished two wooden ducks.

I will try sewing some of his shirt cuff buttons on with elastic thread so that they can remain buttoned. Mr. B. continues to spend one hour per day working on his craft projects. He has completed four link doormats.

I gathered some lumber and made a simple ramp so that he can get down the one step onto a screened porch. He enjoys being out where he can watch the children next door, shoo squirrels from the bird feeder, admire his apple tree and wave to the neighbors. Mr. B. is getting more independent in dressing his lower extremities. Once his pants are put over his knee he can reach back and pull them up. I have ordered a reaching stick so that he can pick up things off of the floor without danger of tipping over his wheel chair.
Susan Maertz, COTA[27]
Founder of Supportive Care Service
St. Paul, MN

Voluntary Health Agency

I plan and supervise both the recreation and water-therapy programs for a chapter of the Multiple Sclerosis Society. The recreation program includes activities of daily living, socialization, arts and crafts, grooming, entertainment, outings to such places as restaurants, museums, the aquarium and a play. Annual events include a luncheon for 200 members and a small group outing on the "Floating Hospital." My staff includes a recreation assistant and two part time recreation aides.

The water therapy program (shown in Figure 11-2), considered by many physicians to be the most beneficial form of therapeutic exercise, is provided at five different community-based wheelchair-accessible pools in different locations to serve the wide location of members. Participants are able to increase their flexibility, range of motion, muscle tone and physical independence. I send letters to new members telling them about the benefits and inviting them to participate.

The weekly/recreation groups are also scheduled in five different locations and service primarily the moderately to severely disabled, including the homebound. Many times people who are homebound lose contact with the outside world. The programs give people a chance to get out of their homes, participate in exercise, table games and crafts, and develop and strengthen hand-eye coordination. The programs actually meet each day, but in a different location. I've also had OTA students participate in both programs.

My job is creative, rewarding, and gratifying. It provides for a varied experience which is hectic at times, but allows for an opportunity to work with various populations in different settings.

Geraldine Williams, COTA
Director of Recreation Activities
Multiple Sclerosis Society

Pet Facilitated Therapy

Supportive therapy is a major part of an occupational therapy assistant's job. Animals can become an excellent tool for this type of therapy, and I have found a pet therapy program can be beneficial to the staff as well as the patients. I now work as a COTA in a nursing care center. From day one at my new job, I talked about pet therapy to anyone who would listen. First, we established a plan for pet therapy, all department heads were consulted, and input was gathered from each one. Rules were laid out regarding where the pets would stay in the facility. Then, the selection of pets began.

One of my patients exhibited signs of depression. Heidi, the dog and I started visiting her. Heidi sat by the patient and treated her like she was the most important person in the world. Then Princess the rabbit was brought and allowed to sit on the patient's lap when I was present. And after about two weeks, the patient changed. First she asked me to help her get dressed. Then, one day she was waiting for Heidi and me at the front door of the facility saying "Heidi loves me—she really does."

Another patient really liked birds. When she was weak and disoriented following an illness, I took Blue Boy the parakeet to visit her. While I sat on the side of the bed he was perched on my finger as we talked—first about Blue Boy then about previously enjoyed subjects. Although she talked a little and kept watching the bird who was by that time on my shoulder, I was discouraged.

However, that afternoon, her daughter said "Mom was so excited about that parakeet, she wants to come down to see him."

Patient awareness and increased interaction between staff and patients make all the work involved in carrying out a pet therapy program worthwhile.

Diane Rush, COTA/L
Norworth Convalescent Center

Contract COTA

I'm a "temp" a "pool person," a "contract COTA." In short, I work for contract agencies and I love it. I never know just what I'll find when I walk in the door of a new placement. Since the time allotted for my orientation is usually one to three minutes, I've got to learn fast, take good notes, and keep cool. Each situation holds a new challenge.

A spirit of adventure, a knowledge of relaxation techniques and a familiarity with basic mechanics are definite assets. The fact that I'm "here today and gone tomorrow" puts me in the unique position of being able to offer respite to the over-stressed regular staff, and they are usually delighted to allow me that privilege. My patients are the extra-challenging individuals.

When the work is available, the money is good. Working for several agencies is a mixed blessing: more work, less play; more money, less freedom. I don't get paid for personal days, sick days, holidays or vacations.

The easy part is that when the going gets tough, I often get going, along to the next assignment. The hard part is that by the time I begin to feel comfortable in a situation, the crisis is over, the census is down, or a new permanent employee is hired, and I am history. I may have worked with Mrs. Jones for a while and helped her begin to work through her denial, anger and bargaining, but I probably will miss out on the acceptance part of the process. Mr. Brown can dress himself now and is beginning to get some return in that left arm, but it's unlikely that I'll be around to see him at work with somebody new, just when we were really beginning to know each other. All of this has taught me that the ties I make will soon be broken.

If nothing else, temporary work has made me a realist. I avoid the problems that don't concern me and handle the ones that do, all the while feeling grateful for the little gifts and small successes.

Now that I've done it both ways, which is really better—agency work or a "real" job? To me, it's kind of like choosing a mate. You pick the qualities that are important and the set of problems you think you can live with; then you enjoy one and make the best of the other. At its worst, agency work is stressful and uncertain. At its best, it is creative and liberating. Always, I find it demanding, broadening and enriching, and right now, that's enough for me.

Mary E. Haas, COTA
Spectrum Temporary Services
Milwaukee, Wisconsin
Condensed from OT for Sale or Rent, *OT Forum*, 1989.

SUGGESTIONS

1. Be alert to new areas of practice mentioned in job announcements, as topics of presentation at conferences or in publications.
2. Find out about occupational therapy assistants in unique roles and settings in your part of the country.
3. Contact a local occupational therapy assistant program to find out the variety of placements of recent and earlier graduates.

READING OBJECTIVES

1. Identify newly developing areas for occupational therapy assistant practice.
2. Give examples of positions filled by occupational therapy assistants which may not require that specific training.
3. List types of non-traditional roles and settings served by occupational therapy assistants.

REFERENCES

[27]Excerpts from COTA Concerns column *Occupational Therapy News*.

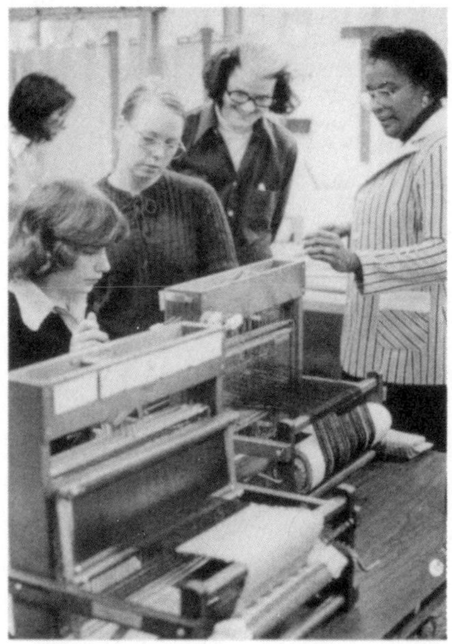

Figure 11-1: In the role of faculty member in an occupational therapy assistant college curriculum, the occupational therapy assistant supervises students learning weaving as a therapeutic activity. A visiting counselor learns that weaving may be done on upright frames or floor looms and table looms as well as off-loom, that it is used therapeutically for both the physically disabled and those with psychosocial dysfunction, and that it is particularly effective in meeting goals which involve perception and cognitive or learning skills.

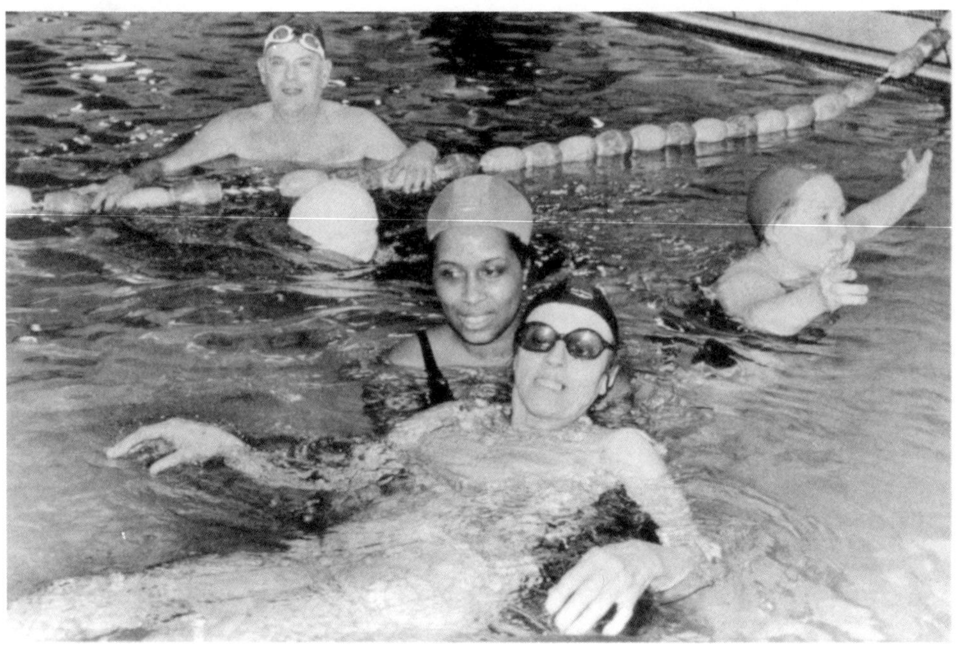

Figure 11-2: As supervisor of the Water Therapy Program, the occupational therapy assistant not only arranges for volunteers and occupational therapy assistant students to participate at times but does so as well. Here she supports a member so that she can gain the benefits of movement in the water. Photo credit: Michael Paras, 1984 for The Multiple Sclerosis Society.

PART III

BEYOND THE CLINICAL SETTING: THE OCCUPATIONAL THERAPY ASSISTANT AS A HEALTH PROFESSIONAL

CHAPTER 12

CREDENTIALING

NATIONAL CERTIFICATION

A graduate of an occupational therapy assistant training program which is approved by the American Occupational Therapy Association (AOTA) is eligible for certification by the American Occupational Therapy Certification Board (AOTCB). The certification examination is offered twice each year in January and July and is administered by Assessment Systems Inc. It consists of 250 multiple choice questions and allows 4 hours for completion. Upon advance request it may be administered in most states of the U.S. and in foreign countries as well. Applicants who cannot take the examination on Saturday for religious reasons may request Sunday administration. Requests for special needs must be made well in advance.

After the OTA Program Director sends a list of those eligible they receive applications for the exam and an instruction booklet with sample questions. The application must be returned with a fee by the stated deadline. Many schools offer test taking preparation materials or workshops. Applicants are notified two weeks prior to the exam of the testing site. A weighted scoring system is used.

Participants will receive notification of their results. If the examination was passed successfully, the individual will be offered the opportunity to apply for certification by the American Occupational Therapy Association which will entitle the use of the initials COTA after the occupational therapy assistant's name. COTA refers to the national certification designation–certified occupational therapy assistant. The school receives a composite of the scores for all applicants from that school. Individual scores will not be provided to the school. Names of all those who passed the exam are published in the *American Journal of Occupational Therapy*. Graduates who did not pass the exam may reapply directly to the testing agency to retake the exam. There is no limit to the number of times the exam may be retaken.

The approved insignia for COTAs is shown in Figure 12-1. It is oval, red, white and blue and includes both COTA and certified occupational therapy assistant.

Procedure for National Certification

1. Complete all academic requirements for an AOTA approved educational program for the occupational therapy assistant.
2. Complete all fieldwork requirements.
3. Three months prior to the January or July exam obtain an application for the certification examination for occupational therapy assistants.
4. Submit the application and fee by the deadline stated in the application booklet.
5. Successfully complete the examination.
6. File for certification (and AOTA membership if desired).

STATE CREDENTIALING

Credentialing at the state level is separate from national certification and depends on state licensure regulations. By 1989 there were 46 states with Occupational Therapy regulation. In such states only qualified individuals as defined in the legislation may practice occupational therapy or use a title including the words occupational therapy. Table 12-1 lists the states while the Appendix provides full information for each. Figure 12-2 shows the states graphically.

State OT Practice Acts initiated before the national certification examination for occupational therapy assistants was initiated do not require an examination for state certification as an occupational therapy assistant. New York State (NYS), as an example, does not require examination for occupational therapy assistants. (Of course, amendments to the law are possible in the future). NYS Certification is determined by proof of graduation from an approved OTA educational program.

Some foreign trained occupational therapists have sought state certification as occupational therapy assistants if their educational background did not meet the minimum for State licensure at the professional level. However, this may not be possible as State OTA educational requirements must be met. Licensed individuals may choose to so identify themselves. Thus some certified occupational therapy assistants will use COTA/L after their names indicating that they are both licensed in their state and certified nationally.

When enacting licensure a State Board for Occupational Therapy Practice is formed which generally includes occupational therapy personnel and consumer representation. COTAs are represented in some states.

In seeking state credentialing the individual must initiate the process.

Procedure for State Credentialing

1. Write to the State agency for an application and requirements for state credentialing. This should be done prior to graduation, so that it can be submitted immediately thereafter.
2. Arrange for the college or OTA school to send an official transcript to the State office. This usually requires completing and signing a form in the registrar's office and paying a fee for the transcript. This should not be done until all graduation requirements are completed, so that the transcript will verify graduation.
3. Complete the application providing any required photographs and signatures.
4. Mail the completed application and fee to the appropriate State office.

Table 12-2 compares credentialing for one state with national certification.

IN THE WORDS OF AN OCCUPATIONAL THERAPY ASSISTANT

Maryland is one of the states that has a licensing board. The Maryland State Board of Occupational Therapy Practice consists of three OTRs, one COTA (Figure 12-3), a consumer, and a secretary. As the COTA member of the Board, I feel it is important to encourage any COTAs or COTA committees to work closely with their state associations when their licensing board is being formed. It is necessary that much communication be involved so that, by law, a COTA will be a member of their state licensing board. This position can offer a good working relationship between OTRs and COTAs as well as provide visibility and a method of recognition for COTAs as professionals.[28]

Nancy H. Rehmeyer, COTA
Maryland State Board of
Occupational Therapy Practice

SUGGESTIONS

1. Write to your occupational therapy state licensure office or that of a nearby state requesting a copy of the Occupational Therapy Practice Act.
2. Find out the composition of the occupational therapy licensure board and some issues it has encountered.
3. Check with your State occupational therapy association about the status of licensure and potential changes in your state.
4. Write to the American Occupational Therapy Certification Board for its brochure on certification.

READING OBJECTIVES

1. Identify the agency that grants use of the initials, COTA.
2. List the requirements for national certification.
3. Compare state and national credentialing.
4. Explain the meaning of State licensure.

REFERENCES

[28]Adapted from Occupational Therapy News, August 1982.

TABLE 12-1
STATES WITH LICENSURE OR OTHER REGULATORY LAWS COVERING OCCUPATIONAL THERAPY AND THE OCCUPATIONAL THERAPY ASSISTANT BY 1989

Alaska	Missouri
Arizona	Montana
Arkansas	Nebraska
California	New Hampshire
Connecticut	New Mexico
Delaware	New York
District of Columbia	North Carolina
Florida	North Dakota
Georgia	Ohio
Hawaii	Oklahoma
Idaho	Oregon
Illinois	Pennsylvania
Indiana	Puerto Rico
Iowa	Rhode Island
Kansas	South Carolina
Kentucky	South Dakota
Louisiana	Tennessee
Maine	Texas
Maryland	Utah
Massachusetts	Virginia
Michigan	Washington
Minnesota	West Virginia
Mississippi	Wisconsin

TABLE 12-2
COMPARISON BETWEEN STATE AND NATIONAL REQUIREMENTS FOR ONE STATE[1]
NEW YORK STATE VS. AOTA CERTIFICATION

*NYS Certification**	*Similarities*	*AOTA Certification*
Fee covers 3 yrs. ($95 in 1989)	Fee required	Fee for examination ($175 in 1989)
State requirement for OT practice-NYS certified OTA	Certification designation	National recognition-COTA
Associate degree (or 2 yrs. college) required	Completion of approved OTA Program necessary	Associate degree or certificate of completion of shorter programs acceptable
No exam**		Take exam in Jan. or July
Send for application in advance from NYS Department of Education		Application sent after OTA program provides list of eligible students
After graduation submit application to NYS Department of Education	Must submit application	Apply 2 months prior to exam
Submit official transcript verifying actual completion of degree	Verification required	Name must be included on list from school to testing agency indicating expected completion of program.

[1]as of 1989.

*New York State certifies rather than licenses occupational therapy assistants under the Occupational Therapy Practice Act.

**Since the NYS OT Practice Act was enacted prior to the introduction of the AOTA OTA examination no exam was required in the initial implementation of the Practice Act.

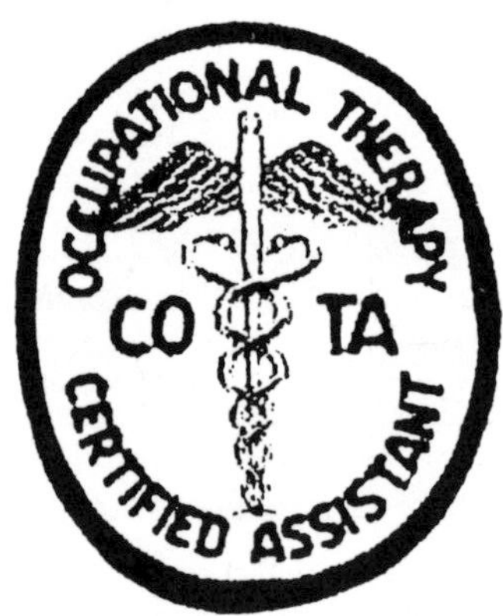

Figure 12-1: Insignia for the certified occupational therapy assistant.

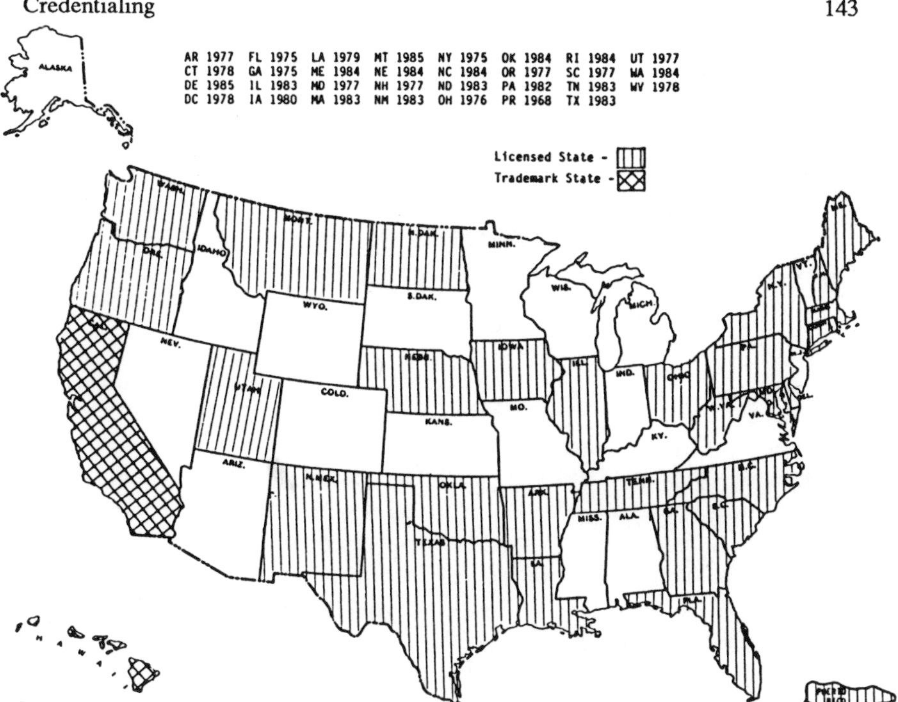

Figure 12-2: State Regulation of occupational therapy. Source: State Regulatory Information Packet, August 1989, AOTA.

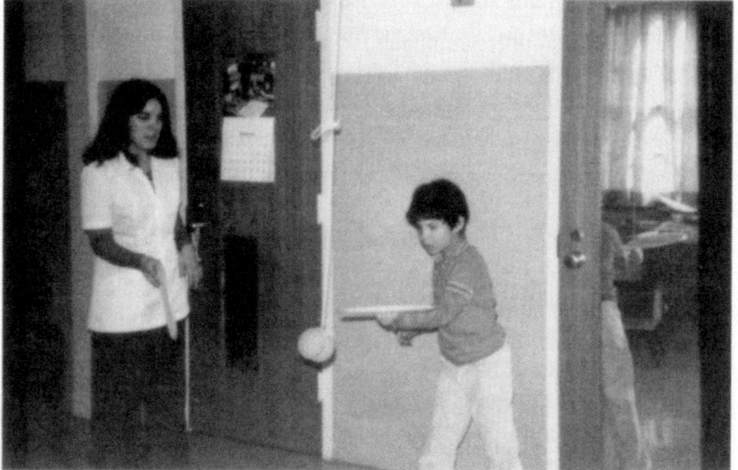

Figure 12-3: The occupational therapy assistant shown in her full time job setting is also a member of her state Occupational Therapy Licensure Board. Here she uses an activity for therapeutic purposes covered under the Occupational Therapy Practice Act.

CHAPTER 13

OCCUPATIONAL THERAPY PROFESSIONAL ORGANIZATIONS

INTERNATIONAL

The World Federation of Occupational Therapists (WFOT) held its first congress in Scotland in 1954. It was founded with 10 member countries. By 1985 there were 33 full or associate member countries. Occupational therapists can be individual professional members, and occupational therapy assistants can be contributing members. WFOT was admitted to the World Health Organization in 1957.

Since educational requirements for occupational therapists vary by country, and many do not require a full baccalaureate college degree; most of the member countries do not have a separate training program for an occupational therapy assistant category. Brazil had a separate training program for occupational therapy assistants, and Barbados had considered introducing a program following the U.S.A. model. In some individual cases U.S. trained occupational therapy assistants with a two year college degree and experience have been accepted for practice in occupational therapy in other countries. A 1984 survey of AOTA members living abroad brought responses from occupational therapy assistants in countries as diverse as Canada, England, Japan, Israel, and West Germany.

The tables which follow list member countries and those that have training programs for occupational therapy technical or support level personnel. The photos show occupational therapy in member countries.

The World Federation of Occupational Therapists (WFOT) holds a World Congress every four years in a member country. As is true of other professional conferences, there are exhibits, speakers, films, business meetings, workshops and social events which provide opportunities for participants to meet one another. Occupational therapy assistants are welcome participants. Site examples: 1974 USA, 1978 Israel, 1982 West Germany.

Member countries have occupational therapy associations while associate members are still forming associations. Countries other than those which are

WFOT members may provide occupational therapy services but do not have an occupational therapy association.

WFOT publishes proceedings in conjunction with the World Congress of Occupational Therapists. A WFOT Bulletin is published as well.

Each member country elects a delegate and alternate to the World Federation of Occupational Therapists. Delegates meet every two years in a Council and circulate regular information to their constituent organization. *Occupational Therapy News* (which as of October 1989 became an insert in AJOT) of the American Occupational Therapy Association publishes a regular WFOT column.

NATIONAL

The American Occupational Therapy Association (AOTA) provides the occupational therapy assistant with an excellent opportunity to participate both as a student and as a practitioner in the national professional organization.

The Association sets standards for the education and practice of occupational therapy assistants and therapists; promotes the field of occupational therapy via the production and distribution of public information materials including films; develops and administers certification examinations and maintains records of those who are certified; publishes the *American Journal of Occupational Therapy* (AJOT), *OT Week*, specialty section newsletters, and special educational materials; carries out recruitment activities; lobbies for legislation relevant to occupational therapists; collects and distributes data on occupational therapy practice and personnel; and provides for forums, conferences and workshops.

The Association recognizes the importance of the occupational therapy assistant and the student and provides for their representation and participation in all facets of the governing structure. The charts which follow show the organizational structure for both the member organization in which people participate on a voluntary basis and the national office with its paid staff.

Every occupational therapy assistant program has three voting members of the AOTA Commission On Education (COE), a faculty member, a field work representative and a student. In addition occupational therapy assistant program representatives are elected proportionately to the COE steering committee.

The official student representative to the AOTA Commission on Practice is elected from an occupational therapy assistant educational program by student members of the Association.

The American Occupational Therapy Association is a member organization with a national office. The certified occupational therapy assistant (COTA) and occupational therapy assistant student are entitled to important membership privileges and rights.

Members of the Association are entitled to vote for representatives and officers of the Association, to serve on committees, to participate in annual conferences and regional meetings, and to join specialty sections. These consist of Developmental Disabilities, Physical Disabilities, Geriatrics, Mental Health, Work Programs, Administration and Management, and Sensory Integration. The Association is an excellent resource and will respond to inquiries by telephone or through the mail. Members receive *AJOT* (including *Occupational Therapy News*) and *OT Week*.

Occupational therapy assistants and students can submit articles, letters or questions to specialty section newsletters, *OT Week*, and *The American Journal of Occupational Therapy*, as well as to other occupational therapy publications.

The American Occupational Therapy Association holds an annual conference in which occupational therapy assistants are active participants. Conferences have presentations on the practice, education and trends of occupational therapy, exhibits of new equipment and books, demonstrations of therapeutic techniques, working sessions on association business, film presentations and many opportunities to informally meet and exchange ideas. Occupational therapy assistants are invited to present papers as well as attend meetings and events.

A COTA representative and alternate were elected as AOTA officers for the first time in 1985. There are COTAs serving on monographs, recognitions, certification, and other committees. Many occupational therapy assistants have held prominent positions in occupational therapy association activities. COTAs may be elected to the Representative Assembly which is the governing body through which representatives from each state vote on policies and documents which if passed become official.

Awards have been established for COTAs at both the national and local level (Figure 13-4). COTAs named to the Roster of Honor are entitled to use the initials ROH after their names. This is comparable to FAOTA for OTRs who are honored by being named Fellows of the American Occupational Therapy Association.

A COTA Task Force was created in 1980 with the specific charge to (1) provide an inventory of perceived COTA needs and (2) suggest ways that the state and national organizations could be responsive to those needs. By 1984 the task force had identified objectives initiated either by the membership or by the task force itself, had acted upon them and offered follow-up as necessary. Examples of objectives and outcomes follow in Table 13-3.

In October 1986 a COTA State Contact survey was conducted, with the COTA advisory committee providing a final report in 1988. Established goals included: (1) To identify marketing strategies to clarify role and function of

COTAs, (2) To examine barriers limiting COTA service delivery and to develop a plan to minimize those barriers, (3) To develop strategies for ongoing development of COTAs and their roles, (4) To promote creative OTR/COTA partnerships, (5) To develop strategies to increase involvement of COTAs at local, state and national levels.

The American Occupational Therapy Foundation (AOTF) was established in 1965. Its purposes include advancing the science of occupational therapy and increasing public knowledge and understanding of occupational therapy. The Foundation is a charitable organization which accepts donations and provides grants to support its purposes.

In the area of research it publishes the "Occupational Therapy Journal of Research" and provides support funding for special projects. In the area of education AOTF offers scholarships and produces flyers and booklets which educate the community to issues related to occupational therapy. It also operates a professional library with items in the collection available through interlibrary loan. In 1989 it announced a plan to promote OT among other professionals.

Annual membership applications from the American Occupational Therapy Association include the opportunity for contributions to AOTF.

The American Student Committee of the Occupational Therapy Association (ASCOTA) was initiated for the purpose of providing a means whereby student members of the American Occupational Therapy Association (AOTA) may effectively contribute to the process of decision making. It also promotes the well-being of students involved in occupational therapy educational programs and enhances their knowledge of the profession. ASCOTA facilitates sharing of ideas, serves as a forum for discussion and serves as a centralized source of information and materials.[28] An ASCOTA newsletter called " 'OT Line" (Figure 13-5) is circulated to students via educational programs.

Each of the elected general directors of the ASCOTA Steering Committee, Chair, Secretary and Fiscal Manager, may be either an occupational therapy assistant (OTA) student or an occupational therapy (OT) student. In addition there are two vice chairs—one representing occupational therapy programs and the other occupational therapy assistant programs. The OTA vice chair serves as the representative of ASCOTA to the AOTA Commission on Practice (COP), as nominating committee chair and as liaison for OTA student concerns and interests. Students who are members of AOTA are eligible to vote and be nominated to run for office in ASCOTA.

Each occupational therapy and occupational therapy assistant educational program selects a delegate to represent students from the program. AOTA student membership fees help to provide funding for a student delegate from each entry level program to attend the annual meeting of ASCOTA during the

AOTA's annual conference. Students must be members of AOTA to participate.

The American Occupational Therapy Political Action Committee (AOTPAC) and The American Occupational Therapy Certification Board (AOTCB), created in 1986, are other national groups linked with the AOTA.

STATE AND LOCAL OCCUPATIONAL THERAPY ASSOCIATIONS

There are 52 state occupational therapy associations including the District of Columbia and Puerto Rico.

In large states such as New York and California there are subdivisions or district associations as well. In addition to occupational therapy assistants and students participating in regular meetings many active organizations have a student unit incorporating both OT and OTA students. The state association may provide student scholarships as well.

Depending on the specific by-laws of the state association COTAs are generally eligible for membership at a reduced rate, may serve on or head committees, and might be elected to serve on the board or in a particular office.

Many state associations have annual conferences at which prominent speakers are featured, exhibits presented, COTA meetings held, and a COTA of the year may be honored. COTAs and OTA students may choose to make presentations and/or operate exhibit booths. Associations with large memberships may hold monthly or quarterly meetings as well and have specialty sections for focused discussions on a particular area of practice. In addition many state and district associations publish and distribute newsletters, which include notification of coming events and may list job openings as well. Attending state association meetings provides participants with a chance to meet other members of the profession, become aware of issues important to occupational therapy, and give input or ideas.

There are occupational therapy councils linking large state or municipal hospital systems, and regional councils have been created to deal with fieldwork placement.

COTAs participate actively in general areas of interest including: public relations, recruitment, job placement, membership, community liaison, and legal issues. Some state associations have a COTA representative position and some have separate COTA groups in addition to providing for general participation.

Many state associations have a job placement service. It may be a listing of positions announced in a newsletter, an actual resource with a COTA coordinating occupational therapy assistant jobs available and COTAs seeking positions, or a mailing of job listings for a fee.

REGIONAL

Cooperative efforts among neighboring states are important for both information sharing when membership in each state is small and to facilitate uniform planning when there is a regular interchange of students.

Regional occupational therapy fieldwork councils have been in existence for many years. These were designed primarily to set procedures and handle scheduling with regard to placement of students in clinical centers for required fieldwork. In many cases responsibilities were expanded with some groups undertaking projects which could be models for national use such as computerized matching of students and placement sites or a comparison of fieldwork objectives for the OTA and OT student. Some occupational therapy fieldwork councils have developed their own manuals on such areas as establishing a fieldwork program or on supervision of students. Some have created standardized forms for requesting or confirming fieldwork sites, for providing individual student data to a center, or for recording observations of a fieldwork center by a faculty member during a site visit. As occupational therapy has expanded, some fieldwork councils have become more localized or have been divided into units covering a single state. Generally they are comprised of representatives from all occupational therapy educational programs with clinical representatives as well.

Regional occupational therapy assistant groups and conferences have evolved as occupational therapy assistants have felt the need to share and meet with one another. Issues are sometimes unique to one region of the country, and national conferences are often too distant for large numbers of COTAs to attend. Thus phenomena such as The Great Southern COTA Conference have been created.

IN THE WORDS OF AN OCCUPATIONAL THERAPY ASSISTANT

Our SOTA (student occupational therapy association) Club at Madison Area Technical College in Madison, WI has been involved in a number of projects this year. A service project was held in July to help buy a piano for a drop-in center for mentally ill people. We carried out this idea with help from the Wisconsin Occupational Therapy Association (WOTA).

Our organization is now raising money to offset the cost of attending the AOTA Conference. Projects will include AOTA calendar sales and a raffle. T-shirts were already sold at our state conference in September. Proclaiming "Total Health through Occupational Therapy," the shirts were designed by one of our students and silkscreened by an entire class.

This fall we are inviting COTAs to speak at our monthly meetings. By

hearing about the thoughts and experiences of these practicing COTAs, we hope to gain a greater understanding of different practice areas and possibilities available to us. However, our first meeting was a student "get acquainted" time during which SOTA, WOTA, and AOTA were explained.[29]
Laurie Huggett, OTA Student
Madison Area Technical College
Wisconsin

SUGGESTIONS

1. When traveling in a WFOT country, visit an occupational therapy department and compare it with those you've already seen in the U.S.
2. Contact The American Occupational Therapy Association at 6000 Executive Blvd., Rockville, MD to request information of a specific or general nature.
3. Learn about scholarships provided by the American Occupational Therapy Foundation and brochures currently available.
4. Find out about the occupational therapy association in your state—meetings, committees, scholarships, job placement service, dues, newsletters, student activities.

READING OBJECTIVES

1. Name and give the initials for the national occupational therapy association and give examples of its services.
2. Name and give the initials for the international occupational therapy association and state how often a Congress is held.
3. Name the occupational therapy organization which accepts tax-deductible contributions and supports occupational therapy research.
4. Give an example of the functions of a state occupational therapy association.
5. Name or give the initials of the organization which serves only occupational therapy or occupational therapy assistant students.

REFERENCES

[28]ASCOTA Reference Handbook for Students and Educators, August 1982.
[29]Adapted from *The 'OT Line*. Vol. VI, No. 1, February 1986.

TABLE 13-1
WORLD FEDERATION OF OCCUPATIONAL THERAPISTS FULL MEMBERS AND ASSOCIATE MEMBERS

Argentina	Kenya
Australia	Malaysia (Associate Member)
Austria	Netherlands
Belgium	New Zealand
Canada	Norway
Chile	Philippines
Colombia	Portugal
Denmark	Singapore (Associate Member)
Federal Republic of Germany	South Africa
Finland	Spain
France	Sweden
Hong Kong	Switzerland
Iceland (Associate Member)	Thailand
India	United Kingdom
Ireland	United States
Israel	Venezuela
Italy (Associate Member)	Zimbabwe (Associate Member)
Japan	

TABLE 13-2
WFOT COUNTRIES WITH RECOGNIZED TRAINING OF SUPPORT STAFF

Country	*Category of Staff*	*Length of Course*	*Qualification*
Western Australia	Mental Health OT Aides	One day per week over five months	Certificate of Training
Denmark	OT Helper	8 months (1059 hrs.)	
Holland	MBO/AT (MAT) MBO/AB	748 hours over 3 yrs. Part time-3 yrs.	MBO/AT
Norway	OT Helper	6–12 months	
South Africa	Technical Instructor	±18 mos. part time	Certificate of Competence & Attendance
Sweden	OT Helper	12–18 months	
Switzerland	Activational Therapist (Restricted to Geriatrics)	18 months	Activational Therapist
United Kingdom	OT Helpers Technicians	6–12 months 36 day release	Certificate of Satisfactory Attendance
United States	Certified OT Assistants	Varies 9–18 months Varies in content	Certified OT Assistant
Venezuela	OT Aide	6 hours per week for 36 weeks	Certificate of Competence
New Zealand (to set up)			

TABLE 13-3
ACTIVITIES OF THE COTA TASK FORCE 1980–1984

Objective (Education)	*Outcome*
1. Better Defined Role Delineation	Role delineation is again in revision.
2. Relevant and affordable Continuing Education for COTAs	Professional Development Office charged to develop a plan.
3. Increase entry level knowledge of structure and function of AOTA	A learning package "A Closer Look at AOTA" was developed.
Objective (Practice)	*Outcome*
1. Define roles of COTA/OTR after entry level.	COTAs are included in Commission on Practice work on subject.
2. Increase information concerning the role of COTAs in Major OT texts.	Letter sent to publisher re: inclusion of COTA information. New textbook being developed.
3. Collect information regarding technical level personnel in other health fields.	Information available through COTA liaison.
Objective (Professional) (Involvement)	*Outcome*
1. Need for COTA advocate at the national level	A COTA liaison appointed in the National Office.
2. Increase COTA involvement in activities of AOTA	COTA participation on commissions and committees has increased.
3. Assure COTA representation on policy making body of AOTA.	COTA Representative at Large to be seated in 1985.
4. Increase COTA contributions to publications.	"COTA SHARE" column developed. Established *Archives*. COTA now on Monograph and Publications Committee.
5. Establish new membership mark for COTAs	Adopted by the Representative Assembly.
6. Increase COTA involvement in conference presentations.	A COTA forum is provided at every annual conference.
7. Establish the Task Force as a standing committee of AOTA	Standard operating procedure developed.
8. Increase number of COTAs choosing *membership* in AOTA versus *Certified Only*.	AOTA Member Services will develop and implement a plan.

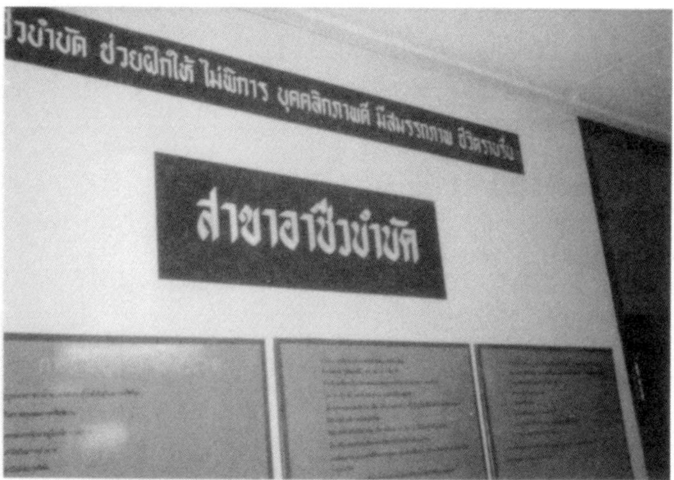

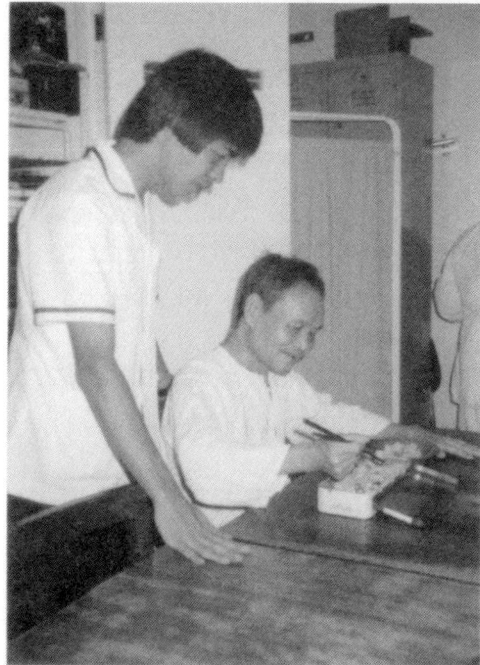

Figures 13-1 & 13-2: The World Federation of Occupational Therapists helps to facilitate communication and exchange visits among therapists from different countries. In these photos by the author the word occupational therapy appears in Thai at the occupational therapy assistant training program in Bangkok, Thailand and an occupational therapy student retrains a patient in the common goal of feeding himself (using chopsticks to transfer squares of foam rubber from box to plate) at Kowloon Hospital, Hong Kong.

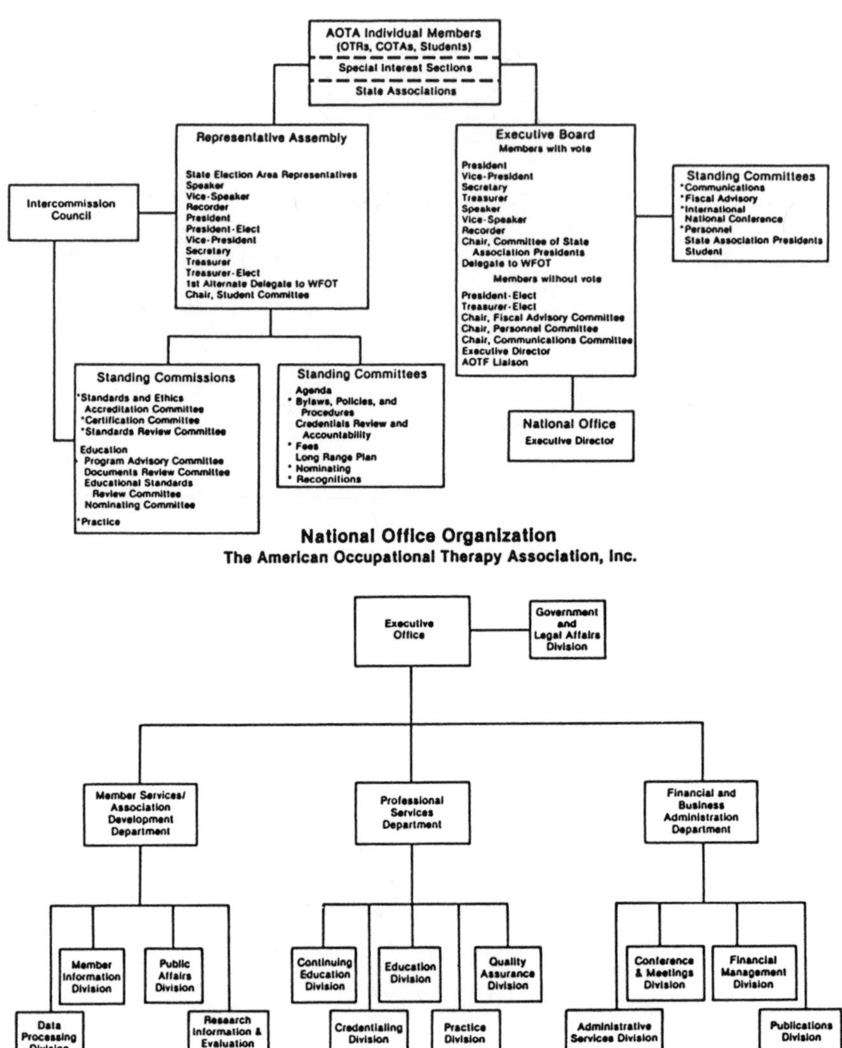

Figure 13-3: Organization Charts of the American Occupational Therapy Association and its national office.

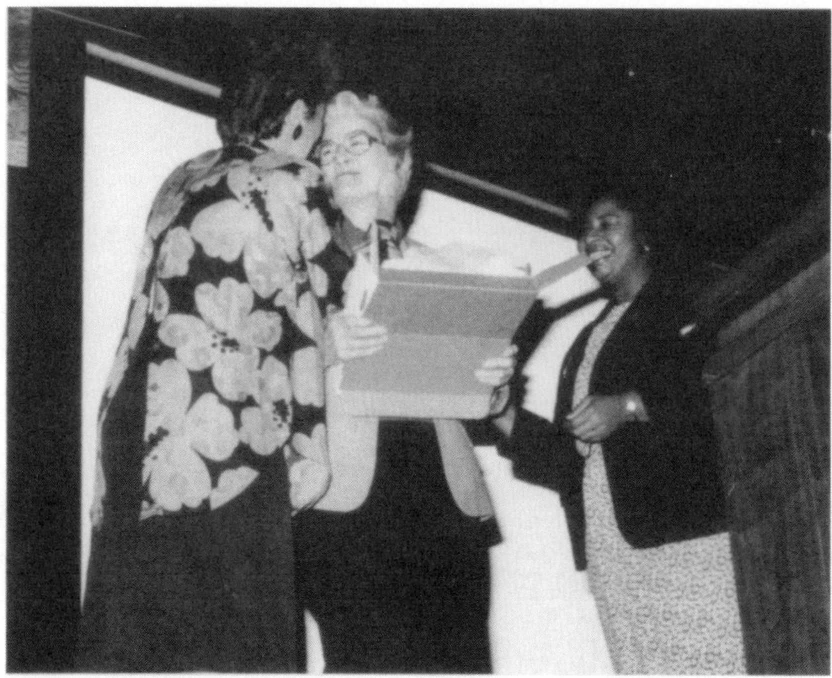

Figure 13-4: Gertrude Pinto, COTA, who had been recognized by her state occupational therapy association as COTA of the Year, receiving an award for her dedication to the occupational therapy assistant as an entity.

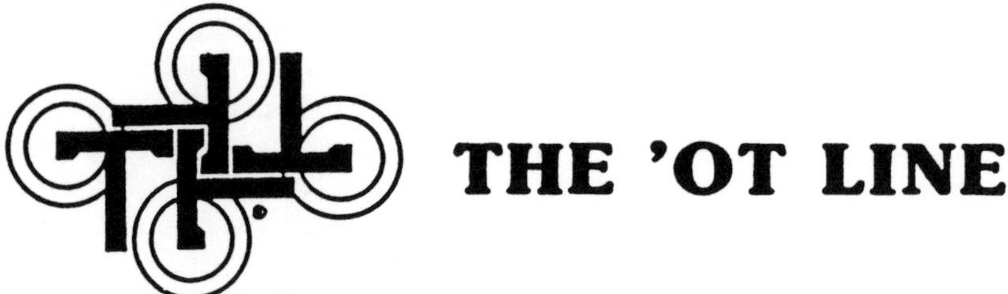

Figure 13-5: The logo for *The 'OT Line*, the newsletter of the American Student Committee of the Occupational Therapy Association, is also the design for an occupational therapy pin sold through the AOTA.

CHAPTER 14

JOB OPPORTUNITIES

JOB OPPORTUNITIES FOR THE OCCUPATIONAL THERAPY ASSISTANT

Expectations

The opportunities for occupational therapy assistants are broad and varied. Traditional areas of employment in hospitals and nursing homes have expanded to community based programs and schools and into non-traditional areas as diverse as demonstration and sales of rehabilitation products and teaching in occupational therapy programs on college campuses. The distribution by state is shown in Figure 14-1.

The Bureau of Labor Statistics and U.S. News & World Report have identified occupational therapy assistants as one of the fastest growing career areas. Jobs are estimated to continue to exceed the supply as shown in Table 14-1.

Sources of Employment Information

With increasing recognition of the occupational therapy assistant there has been an increase in the number of advertisements for COTAs in traditional job sources such as newspapers. However, most new occupational therapy assistants locate positions through placement services offered by the educational programs from which they graduate. Employers seeking COTAs contact occupational therapy assistant programs directly often asking that job announcements be posted, brochures be circulated, or that referrals of graduates be made so that recent graduates can be contacted directly. Table 14-2 lists sources for OT positions.

The American Occupational Therapy Association also provides sources for job market information. There are classified and display advertising sections in both the *American Journal of Occupational Therapy* and in *OT Week*. Job placement sections are featured at annual conferences where participants can record situations wanted, review positions available, and even actually be interviewed during the conference. State and local associations also provide job information.

The newest approach is that of private newsletters created as a business just for the purpose of giving potential employers a way to reach occupational therapists and occupational therapy assistants. In 1985 two such weekly publications were started, "Occupational Therapy Forum" and "Advance." Both are sent free to occupational therapists and occupational therapy assistants and contain job opportunities for COTAs as well as general news about the field. The financial success of these new publications confirms reports that there are more jobs available than personnel to fill them. Students may request free subscriptions.

Types of Positions

Recent advertisements for occupational therapy assistants have included the following types of settings: private special education centers; activities therapy departments; private practice rehabilitation groups; psychiatric centers; long-term care facilities; public schools; mental health and rehabilitation centers; pain programs; programs for industrial injured; skilled nursing facilities; mental rehabilitation units; head injury centers; independent living residences; home therapists associations; pediatric teaching hospitals; and multiple handicapped schools.

Many of the positions available to occupational therapy assistants do not specifically identify COTA in the title. Opportunities that appropriately use the skills of the occupational therapy assistant may be open to others as well. Sometimes this is because there is an anticipation that occupational therapy assistants will not be available or because the employer may not be fully familiar with the training or expertise of occupational therapy assistants or the duties may bridge more than one career. Therefore, occupational therapy assistants need to be alert to and aware of the kinds of opportunities which may best use their skills and attributes. In addition to COTA positions, occupational therapy assistants have been hired into such positions as activity leaders and directors (Figure 14-2), group home counselors, community service workers and other varied positions described in Part II of this book.

Salaries vary by geographic region, type of populations, sponsoring organizations, experience and responsibilities. There are often differences between government civil service salaries and salaries in private institutions. Often salaries are affected by the availability or lack thereof of occupational therapy personnel. Salaries compare very favorably with those for other careers with a similar amount of educational preparation.

Excellent benefit packages are provided in most health care institutions. Government positions generally offer as much as 4 weeks vacation, more than 10 holidays, health insurance, generous sick leave allowance, and education benefits. Services designed to hire and place occupational therapy personnel in changing locations may pay higher salaries by the hour and have more limited benefits. Some are operated by occupational therapists and assistants.

Getting the Job

Knowing that there is a market for OT skills is important. Finding out about specific job openings is a first step; but the most important part to getting a job is selling yourself. Betty Cox, COTA[30] in "How to Apply for a Job on Paper and get the Interview" emphasizes the importance of a resume and cover letter. Many occupational therapy assistants may skip that stage if they are hired by the site where they experienced fieldwork or if they made direct personal contact. However, the interview is essential, and often requires a written resume or an application completed.

The resume should generally be kept to one page which means that persons with considerable experience should choose highlights of their experience, while a person with limited experience might expand on relevant aspects. Essential features of a resume are the name and address, education, and work experience. The latter two should be listed in reverse chronological order with the most recent position or educational experience first. A resume might also include relevant aspects of interests: community activities, additional personal data, professional involvement, and honors or awards. A resume should be typed and well organized although style may vary.

Presenting oneself on paper in some form is usually required prior to fieldwork. Local and regional occupational therapy councils sometimes create a form which all students complete before fieldwork placement. It is reviewed by the potential fieldwork supervisor prior to an interview or the start of fieldwork. It often includes such areas as professional and personal strengths and areas for further development, learning style or preference, experiences desired and special skills.

The interview enables both the interviewer and the interviewee to find out whether they are right for each other. It is a chance for both parties to gain information. When preparing for an interview a number of things should be considered: dress neatly and appropriately; prepare questions to ask about the position; find out some aspects about the center before the interview; bring a resume and/or list of important facts about yourself, including dates and places of employment; and do whatever is best for you to be relaxed and comfortable. Do be prepared to answer questions like, "How would you describe occupational therapy?" and "What do you think the role of an occupational therapy assistant should be in this kind of setting?"

An interview is often required prior to fieldwork placement either for the purpose of selecting from an excess number of applicants and/or to set the stage for a successful experience by clarifying issues in advance and establishing expectations. Some interviews are brief, but most include a tour and opportunity to observe the occupational therapy area. Generally interviews are conducted on a one-to-one basis, but group interviews may be scheduled as well.

Applicants should consider salary, location and responsibilities in selecting a job. The employer will consider experience, availability and skills in selecting an applicant. Both will be interested in whether they would like to work with each other.

IN THE WORDS OF AN OCCUPATIONAL THERAPY ASSISTANT

The COTA education I received is invaluable in running the Activities Department.

Some years ago, during a State Survey, I was accused of doing occupational therapy. The surveyor gave me two choices: (1) Continue directing the Activities Department and get an OTR to do OT, (2) Do OT and get a Director of Activities. Her advice to me was, "Since you are doing such a good job as Director of Activities, why don't you forget you ever went to school and get someone else to do OT."

I took her advice. However, I still continue to do and supervise remedial crafts, passive and active movement, reality orientation and sensory awareness. I just don't document it as OT.

I could not work in physical dysfunction in a hospital; I forgot how to splint. But I cannot forget the philosophy, principles, attitudes and discipline of OT.

It is not just theory—it is a way of life.

Mifa Rogoff
Director of Activities
Bialystocker Home

SUGGESTIONS

1. Look at a "job openings" bulletin board at an occupational therapy assistant educational program or find out how job offers are announced to students.
2. Think about what you would include in your own resume.
3. Contact your state or OT association to learn whether a job placement service exists and review a copy of an OT job newspaper.
4. Ask occupational therapy assistants how they learned about their jobs and why they chose them.
5. Have someone role play an interview with you.

READING OBJECTIVES

1. Discuss expectations regarding the job market for occupational therapy assistants.
2. Identify sources for occupational therapy assistant jobs.
3. State the essential items and possible supplementary items to be included in a resume.
4. List five ways to prepare for an interview.
5. Give examples of factors which may contribute to job selection.

REFERENCES

[30]Cox B, et al: How to Apply for a Job on Paper and get the Interview. AOTA, 1980.

TABLE 14-1
SOURCES FOR OCCUPATIONAL THERAPY ASSISTANT POSITIONS

- Occupational Therapy Assistant Educational Program
  - Office
  - Bulletin Boards
  - Faculty
  - Other students
- Educational Institution (college)
  - Placement Office
  - Career Advisement Center
  - Counseling Office
- Publications
  - General Newspapers
  - American Journal of Occupational Therapy
  - Specialty newspapers such as Occupational Therapy Forum
  - State and local occupational therapy association newsletters
  - OT Week
- Other
  - Fieldwork supervisors
  - Direct contact with clinical settings
  - State and local association job placement services
  - Professional meetings and conferences
    - Direct contact
    - Announcements
    - Posted notices
    - Job placement area
  - General audience services

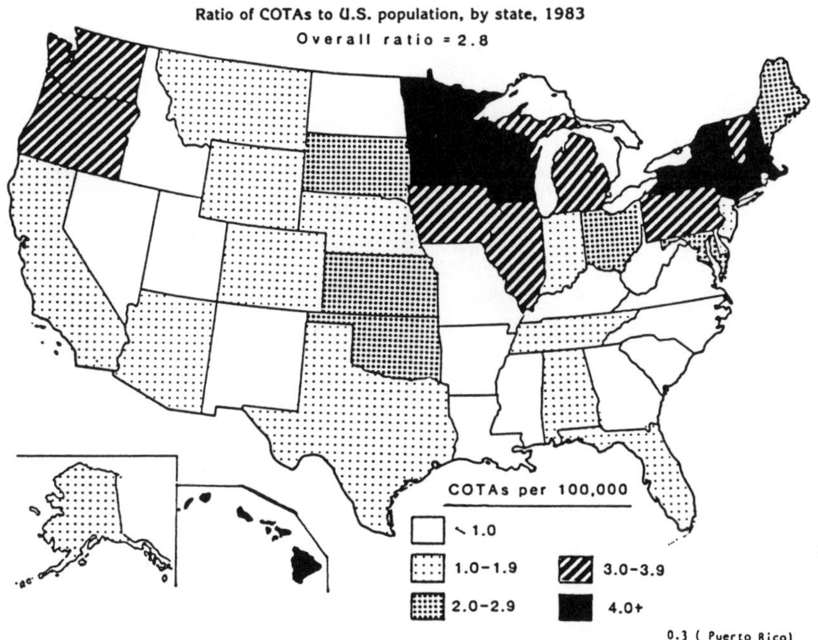

Figure 14-1: Ratio of COTAs to U.S. population, by state, 1983. Source: American Occupational Therapy Association, Occupational Therapy Manpower: A Plan for Progress, 1985.

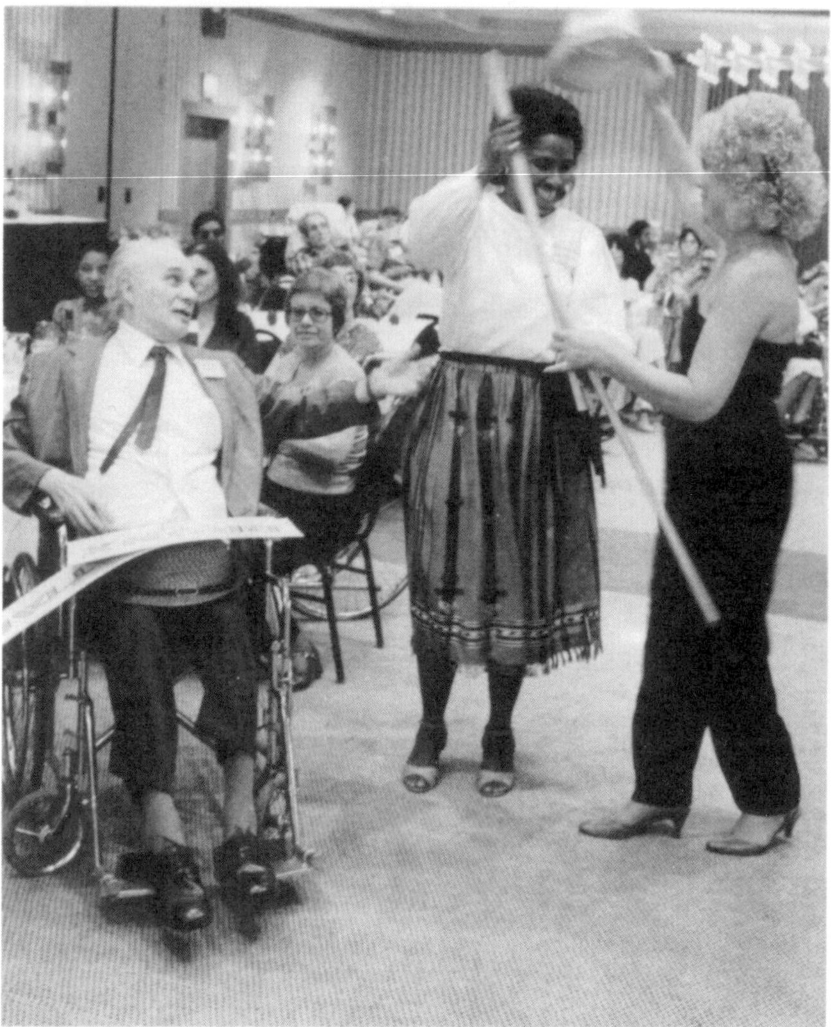

Figure 14-2: This photo shows an occupational therapy assistant in the job title of Activities Director. Approved occupational therapy assistant educational programs are required to include content on managing an activities program. Responsibilities include arranging for entertainment and sometimes even joining the show, as shown.

CHAPTER 15

CONTINUING EDUCATION

CONTINUED LEARNING FOR PROFESSIONAL DEVELOPMENT

A graduate of an occupational therapy assistant program has several options. Most graduates immediately seek a position as an occupational therapy assistant. Others choose to continue full-time education toward a baccalaureate degree. For both of these groups there is also the option of continued supplementary education including reading professional literature, attendance at professional conferences, seminars, and workshops or courses in specialty areas, and in-service training programs. Such continuing education opportunities as shown in Table 15-1 serve to enhance the general training of the occupational therapy assistant and prepare the OTA for more advanced and specialized applications of skills in the clinical setting. Workshops and meetings are usually scheduled at times when they can be taken advantage of by full-time students or full-time employees. OTAs may choose to pursue a bachelor's degree in a related area such as special education, orthotics, or gerontology. They may utilize the knowledge and degree for further specialization in conjunction with occupational therapy assistant practice or as the basis for further education toward a master's degree in occupational therapy.

Some large health care facilities offer college courses directly on site. Such courses are often offered at reduced rates with shorter class times. Each course is in itself useful for enhancing knowledge and may also be credited toward an ultimate degree whether in occupational therapy or a related area. Occupational therapy assistants may choose to move ahead within a specialty area without specifically focusing on occupational therapy. Occupational therapy assistants have earned baccalaureate and advance degrees including masters and doctoral degrees in social work, anthropology, vocational rehabilitation, education, health care administration, counseling, community health, psychology and other majors. In 1986 more than 20% of COTAs were pursuing additional degrees.

The primary area for advanced degrees pursued by occupational therapy assistants is occupational therapy for which there are entry level programs at both the bachelor's degree and master's degree levels.

DECIDING TO BECOME AN OCCUPATIONAL THERAPIST

For occupational therapy assistants interested in becoming occupational therapists the only current approach is by entering an accredited educational program.

Many occupational therapy training programs have attempted to provide specific opportunities for COTAs to build on the occupational therapy knowledge and skills they have already gained in their OTA curricula. Dominican College, for example, started a weekend program to which only occupational therapy assistants could be admitted. Courses meet once every three weeks for a full weekend thus allowing working occupational therapy assistants to continue their education. The first weekend OT program was started at the College of Saint Catherine. Several universities, such as the University of Kansas and the City University of New York have both occupational therapy and occupational therapy assistant programs. This generally allows for a greater ease of transferring credits from one program to the other. There are some students who start out in occupational therapy programs and transfer to occupational therapy assistant programs, but more often the situation is the reversed.

The Wiscouncil, a group representing occupational therapy educational programs and fieldwork centers in Wisconsin, undertook a Career Laddering Project for the Commission of Education of the American Occupational Therapy Association. It reported that by 1982 almost half of the educational programs for occupational therapists had developed specific mechanisms to facilitate the entry of occupational therapy assistants into their curricula. The American Occupational Therapy Association prepares a list of "Non Traditional Options in Entry-Level Professional Programs." It lists programs which offer: 1) alternative class schedules including weekend, evening, self-paced and part-time schedules; and 2) special considerations for course work including proficiency to wave prerequisites or courses, portfolio review, recognition of educational experiences such as workshops, seminars or correspondence study, college level examination program (CLEP) and fieldwork modification.

The Wiscouncil Career Laddering Project report also indicated that in the 5 year period ending in 1982 almost 80% of the educational programs for the occupational therapist had admitted occupational therapy assistants. The report identified the following reasons occupational therapy assistants chose to enter such a program:

Career advancement
Increased independence & responsibilities
Increased pay
Pay preferences
Increased theoretical background

In the same period 100 students transferred from programs for the occupational therapist to occupational therapy assistant programs. Their main reasons were:

Quicker entry into the field
Less investment in education
Increased emphasis on doing versus theory
Role preference
More supervision/less responsibility
More career versus liberal arts emphasis

An alternative program had existed for COTAs to become OTRs. The Career Mobility Plan had provided a procedure for COTAs who had worked for four years in the field to complete a self assessment, enter supervised fieldwork experience for training toward an entry level occupational therapist and subsequently sit for the national certifying examination. This program was phased out and discontinued. As state licensure expanded it was found that the career mobility option, although enabling the initials OTR to be used after the name, did not always allow the COTA who became an OTR to practice as an occupational therapist. Some states required a minimum of a baccalaureate degree in occupational therapy in order to be eligible for professional licensure.

Occupational therapy assistant programs provide information on career laddering in general and usually have information available on specific requirements for admission to educational programs for the occupational therapist in the same geographical area. There may be actual articulation agreements between the schools.

Admission requirements to an OT program might include a set number of liberal arts credits, courses such as statistics, sociology or chemistry, and a minimum grade point average. An occupational therapy assistant student considering continuing education toward becoming an occupational therapist might choose to take courses which may be required on transfer, as elective courses while completing the occupational therapy assistant curriculum. Therefore, it is wise to explore such options well in advance of transfer. Sometimes greater acceptance of credits is achieved once the associate degree and/or COTA is earned. However, students considering transferring may do so prior to completion of an occupational therapy assistant program. It is generally recommended that the occupational therapy assistant work in the field first before deciding to enter an educational program for the occupational therapist.

WAYS TO ENHANCE KNOWLEDGE

There are many ways in which the occupational therapy assistant may expand knowledge after graduation. As the field of occupational therapy has grown so have the number of occupational therapy publications. In addition to the journals and newsletters published by OT professional organizations, there are additional journals focusing on occupational therapy in specialty areas. These include the *Occupational Therapy Journal of Research, Occupational Therapy in Mental Health, Physical and Occupational Therapy in Geriatrics*, and *Occupational Therapy in Health Care*. Occupational therapy periodicals are listed in Table 15-2. New and revised volumes are constantly being added to the literature. Relevant literature may actually name occupational therapy in the title or relate to it with regard to types of patients or clients treated in settings in which occupational therapy services are provided. Reading or reviewing such literature enhances awareness of the field.

Continuing education enables a COTA to keep up with new developments. In addition to reading, workshops, conferences or formal courses the variety of professional association learning opportunities for COTAs is growing.

As the number of COTAs increases, a need for discussion has led to organized and announced gatherings around common interests. For example, one group of COTAs met to discuss the topic, "Where do we go from here?" Presentations included: opportunities for part-time or weekend schooling while working as a COTA, developing expertise in a specialty area with a mentor approach, and providing recognition within the OTA community.

Finding continuing educational opportunities takes awareness and interest. Professional organizations include listings of continuing education opportunities in their newsletters. Such listings include educational program announcements by occupational therapists and occupational therapy assistants, by occupational therapy organizations, and by private companies and individuals who believe their programs are relevant to occupational therapy. Occupational therapy assistants who are members of OT or non-OT professional groups will be notified of conferences and other educational programs sponsored by them. In addition professional organizations often sell or offer the use of their membership lists to groups or individuals wishing to promote an educational program or activity. In such a case an occupational therapy assistant might receive a separate announcement of a continuing education opportunity in the mail.

Another source of continuing education opportunities is bulletin boards. Many health care settings and schools have bulletin boards with announcements for staff and students. Sometimes announcements are sent directly to the facility. At other times an individual will post an announcement that might be appropriate for other staff. Thus, for example, an occupational therapy assistant might learn of a social work or rehabilitation conference that might fulfill an important continuing education need.

The types of continuing educational opportunities vary. Scheduled activities include national, state and local conferences, workshops, seminars, lectures, forums, films, panel presentations, discussion groups, demonstrations, book

CHAPTER 16

ETHICAL AND LEGAL CONSIDERATIONS

INTRODUCTION

There is an increasing awareness of ethical considerations in the health field. Bioethics committees are being established in health care institutions, and daily newspapers carry articles covering government intervention and court decisions regarding individual questions of ethics related to health.

What is health? The World Health Organization's definition includes psychological, physical and social components. All of these must be considered when dealing with moral aspects of the delivery of health care. There are many issues involved. It is important for occupational therapy assistants to recognize the issues and their own moral responsibilities as health professionals. The issues selected for this chapter are autonomy, confidentiality, truth telling, life and death issues, research on human subjects, allocating scarce resources, informed consent, and codes of professional conduct.

AUTONOMY

Autonomy is a fundamental concept which relates to respect for persons. It may refer to the separation of the patient or client from the health professional or the basic idea of "personhood." What constitutes a human being? Does a child have its own autonomy as a person and individual and thus entitlement to treatments; or is the child with a disability subject to the wishes of the parents or the health professional? At the other end of the life continuum, do an older person's wishes regarding treatment and discharge take paramount consideration or should children make the decision for the older adult? Likewise, is the patient considered when a treatment procedure is being thought of, or does the health care worker proceed without regard to how the patient may want the situation handled? Can a health professional enforce a regimen on a patient or is it the patient's right to refuse to participate or receive treatment? To be autonomous, individuals should be allowed to participate as self-determining agents, to be both free of external control and in control of their own affairs or destiny as long as those actions produce no serious harm to other persons. However, some persons cannot act autonomously because they are immature, incapacitated, ignorant, or coerced; for example, children and institutionalized populations such as the profoundly mentally retarded.

The occupational therapy assistant, unlike many other health workers does not "do to the patient" by, for instance, injecting medication, but rather enables patients to "do for themselves." Thus the occupational therapy assistant must consider the rights of the patient and at the same time use the skills learned during training to motivate the patient to make the extra efforts necessary to achieve the goal. The patient or client is still an autonomous individual who may or may not follow through on the proposals presented by the occupational therapy assistant.

CONFIDENTIALITY

Historical Perspectives

There is a long history of medical confidentiality in codes of professional ethics. Hindu medicine mentions the obligations of medical secrecy as does the Hippocratic Oath.

Current Requirements

The *Patient's Bill of Rights* published by the American Hospital Association reads: "The patient has the right to expect that all communications and records pertaining to his care should be treated as confidential." Each health profession has a code including a pledge to preserve confidentiality of the patient's record.

The *Occupational Therapy Code of Ethics* approved by the American Occupational Therapy Association in 1988 includes the statement:

> "The individual shall protect the confidential nature of information gained from educational, practice, and investigational activities unless sharing such information could be deemed necessary to protect the well-being of a third party."

Legal Aspects

There are two kinds of legal protection for medical confidentiality. Positive protection refers to legal actions against professionals who reveal confidential information about their patients. Negative protection is provided by laws which maintain that communications between the health professional and patient is privileged information which the health professional is not required to normally reveal to a court.

Justification

Why is medical confidentiality important?

1. Long-term consequences:
   The promise of confidentiality allows patients to share fully information which may help in their health care.
2. Respect for the rights of patients:
   The general right of privacy is a basic human right.

Counter Argument (Exceptions)

1. Maintaining confidentiality might conflict with the protection of the patient. In the case, for example, of a potential suicide the health professional might have to consider maintaining the secret vs. saving the patient's life.
2. Confidentiality may conflict with the right of an innocent third party, as in the requirement in most states that child abuse cases must be reported to the appropriate government agency.
3. There may be a conflict with the rights and interests of society in general such as, the need to report a contagious disease or a problem such as epileptic attacks that may be dangerous in the person's occupation.

Other Considerations

The increasing number of allied-health personnel in medical care means a greater number of persons having access to medical records of patients.

Computerized health data systems might open access to those who manage the system and who are not covered by a professional code of ethics. A comprehensive file includes a greater amount of data which might be more damaging if confidentiality is violated.

The question of patient access to one's own record becomes important where lifetime records may be stored, and outdated information could be misleading. Such access might be arranged through an intermediary.

Actual Student Case Example

An occupational therapy assistant student completing her internship at a rehabilitation hospital casually mentioned to her mother the name of a patient at the hospital. Her mother in turn shared this in a subsequent telephone conversation with a friend who lived in the geographical area of the patient. This ultimately resulted in the patient's girl friend finding out about his hospitalization which he was trying to keep from her.

Guidelines for Occupational Therapy Assistants and Students

All case studies, treatment plans, evaluations and other patient/client related materials presented to an instructor or to a class or seminar must not carry the patient's name. The entire name may be obliterated or a copy made without the name. The patient's/client's initials or first name only may be used.

Patient's or client's names should not be used in any oral presentations or discussions outside of the clinical setting even with classmates.

Study the *Occupational Therapy Code of Ethics.*

Questions

Why should an occupational therapy assistant be concerned about confidentiality?

In what case might an occupational therapy assistant share a patient's secret with the supervisor?

Is it proper to share a patient's or client's name with an instructor and students in a school seminar?

TRUTH TELLING, LYING AND THE RIGHT TO INFORMATION

Historical Perspectives

The early Hippocratic principle that no harm should be done to patients has been thought to include the concept of not revealing their conditions too starkly to patients. Although other ethical principles are covered in early codes, truth telling is absent from virtually all codes as it was considered important, but not when it endangered the patient. The only early example was in 1568 by a Jewish Physician, Omatus Luisitanus.

Current Requirements

Current professional codes emphasize the "self-determination of clients" indicating that the person be given the information necessary for making informed judgments. Although a child might be too young to give legal consent, the child might be old enough to question a procedure.

The American Hospital Association's *Patient's Bill of Rights* states that the patient has the right to obtain from his physician information concerning diagnosis, treatment and prognosis. The American Medical Association leaves the matter up to the physician. Occupational therapy assistants may find themselves in a position where a patient should be referred back to the physician for information regarding diagnosis or prognosis (expected outcome).

Legal Aspects

The law permits physicians to withhold information from patients where it would clearly hurt their health, but this has been limited by the courts.

The moral and legal rights of clients may differ under state laws, but it is the duty of the health professional to be aware of laws for the particular state and to uphold them. The 1974 Federal Privacy Act also relates to this issue.

Reasons for Truth Telling

The patient's right to know.

The physician's obligation to tell.

Lying or intentional deception threatens the relationship and undermines trust and cooperation. Some hold that except where patients do not want the truth, suppression of truth violates a patient's rights and violates fundamental duties of the professional.

Counter Arguments

1. Truthfulness is impossible
2. Patients do not want bad news
3. Truthful information harms them

Where risks of harm from not telling are low and benefits of not telling the patient substantial, the health professional may legitimately lie, deceive, or underdisclose especially when knowing the facts might induce a negative psychological reaction of a patient.[32]

The physician's choice to lie increasingly involves allied health workers such as occupational therapy assistants who may have to act a part they find neither humane nor wise.

In studies made of patients desire to know, 80% of those asked, indicated that they would want to be told the truth even if their prognosis was bad.

Other Considerations

The central issue is the limits of justified deception and nondisclosure. Sissela Bak[33] states "The art of believing what and how much information should be provided is part and parcel of the therapeutic process."

Although concealment, evasion, and withholding of information may at times be necessary, the burden of proof must rest with those who advocate it.

Case Example

After a series of tests a patient is diagnosed as having terminal inoperable cancer. The physician tells the therapist who has been treating the patient not to disclose this information as, years ago, the patient said that he would not want to know. Some days later the patient says to the therapist, "Every one seems to be very secretive. You're my friend, can you tell me what's wrong with me?" What should the therapist do?

Guidelines

1. Refer requests for direct revelations of diagnosis or prognosis to the physician.
2. Within the patient's ability to comprehend, share information with the patient about the treatment being carried out in occupational therapy and its goals.
3. Try to stall to consult with the supervisor regarding controversial situations in which the occupational therapy assistant must decide whether to reveal or not to reveal information.

Questions

1. Why is it preferable to share information with the patient or client when it will not be harmful?
2. If the patient/client asks about diagnosis or prognosis how might the occupational therapy assistant respond?
3. In what cases might it be appropriate to withhold information from the patient/client?

LIFE AND DEATH ISSUES

Beauchamp[34] emphasizes that humanity or the concept of human life may be identified by genetic characteristics that distinguish it from nonhuman species. A life that is distinctively human includes the ability to use symbols, to imagine, to love, and to perform intellectual skills. Conditions for being a person have included consciousness, self-consciousness, freedom to act on one's own reason, capacity to communicate with other persons, and the capacity to make moral judgments.

Does the institutionalized older adult who may not be responsive lose the status of personhood? There are important ethical issues in the treatment of living persons who are seriously or terminally ill. Words and phrases used include "death with dignity," "euthanasia," "the prolongation of life," "allowing to die," and "mercy killing."

In the Baby Jane Doe case, Baby Jane Doe was found to have spina bifida and hydrocephalus. With treatment to minimize the deformities she could possibly live into her 20s. Without treatment she might live only two years. Does the fact that the infant is disabled make the infant less of a person? Following the legal battle she was actually treated in occupational therapy.

The American Medical Association's guide indicates that the cessation of treatment is considered to be justified only when there is irrefutable evidence that biological death is imminent, and then only extraordinary means may be withheld. Hospitals have systems designating which patients should and should not be resuscitated based on prognosis. In some religious views the adult who is suffering and indicates that he or she cannot bear further surgery or similar procedures may be allowed to refuse such treatment even though it may prolong life. However, in the case of the individual who cannot express wishes such as the infant, it is possible that that person can tolerate the medical condition and would choose to live and as an autonomous person should be given the opportunity of medical intervention.

The term "euthanasia," derived from the Greek, means "good death." It has come to be defined as either painlessly putting to death or failing to prevent death from natural causes in terminal illness. The California Natural Death Act draws a distinction between euthanasia and either refusing treatment or allowing to die. Occupational therapy assistants might have to face such issues not only when working in a hospice program for the dying but in other areas as well.

Life and death decisions might be looked at from the point of view of the health professional. What are the obligations to the dying patient? However, they might also be considered from the point of view of the competent adult. Under what circumstances does a patient have the right to request termination of life? This is the dilemma presented in the play and movie "Who's Life is it Anyway" about a young adult with a spinal cord injury, the kind of patient treated frequently by occupational therapy assistants.

In the case of infants and other incompetent individuals, decisions must be made by parties other than the patients themselves. Ethics committees are increasingly being established in hospitals. During the 1960s the policy of maximal treatment was followed. However, as technology becomes increasingly sophisticated and perinatal nurseries a reality more court cases are being considered.

The difficult question of the appropriate role of health professionals must be considered individually. Should the therapist intervene when knowing that a patient could be trained to become functionally independent through rehabilitation but for whom no treatment is ordered because of a family decision to withhold medical intervention?

Guidelines

Although an occupational therapy assistant may have particular religious persuasions or strong feelings about a given case, professional responsibility must not be compromised. The student should share questions and concerns with the supervisor and may seek guidance where direct involvement is necessary.

RESEARCH ON HUMAN SUBJECTS

Fantastic advances have been made by medical science, many of which have relied heavily on research on human subjects. Recently, however, questions have been raised about risks involved in achieving the benefits offered by science and technology.

Codes of ethics and a committee approach have worked well in highlighting difficult ethical issues and in raising the awareness of those engaged in research. Gorovitz[35] emphasizes the importance of groups such as The National Commission for the Protection of Human Subjects of Biomedical and Behavioral Research for dealing with such moral issues. The AOTA code in relation to evaluation and research reads "Occupational Therapists must use accepted scientific methodology...protect the rights of subjects...have the responsibility to provide explanations...unless as in some...settings there is an explicit exception agreed upon in advance." COTAs are increasingly participating in quality assurance studies.

Historical Perspective

With the close of World War II, when the experiments conducted by Nazi doctors upon the concentration camp inmates were revealed to the world, the medical profession sought to prevent a recurrence of those atrocities by establishing a code of ethics for research on humans. The first such code was the Nuremburg Code of 1949; an updated version of which is the widely cited Declaration of Helsinki of 1964.

Guidelines

An occupational therapy assistant who is asked to have patients participate in a research study should be sure that informed consent has been obtained.

Studies which may cause harm or prevent the patient from receiving appropriate treatment should not be pursued by the occupational therapy assistant.

Questions

How does medical experimentation relate to studies which determine whether quality care is being given in occupational therapy?

What kinds of research on human subjects might be carried out in occupational therapy?

In considering one such study, what ethical guidelines should be established?

ALLOCATING SCARCE RESOURCES

The provision of medical services raises various problems that call for the application of principles of justice. There is first of all the question of how medical resources, for example, manpower, skills, and technology, at all levels of care should be distributed among the citizens of a democracy. Should this matter be determined by the operation of a free marketplace? By some form of utilitarian calculation? Should it be determined by income, by social worth or by proclaiming an equal right to health care for every person irrespective of income, geographical location, or social services rendered? Who should receive medical assistance in those special circumstances where there are not enough resources to go around? Criteria to govern the fair allocation of scarce resources must be decided. Since the number of patients in need may, for example, exceed the number of wheelchairs available, selection will have to be made. "Likelihood of success" tests have been used. Controversial social worth factors include the number of dependents the applicant has or the probable value of future contributions by the applicant to the public good. In occupational therapy such decisions may not be life threatening but none the less require some decision making. Some occupational therapy departments have wait lists for providing such services as hand splints.

Guidelines

If there is a shortage of supplies, time, space, or equipment, consult the supervisor as to which patients or clients take priority.

Questions

Can the occupational therapy assistant be considered a scarce resource?

What kinds of allocation decisions might the occupational therapy assistant have to face?

How might they be handled?

INFORMED CONSENT

The issue of informed consent is a relatively new one in the area of medical ethics. It refers to the health professional giving information before asking the patient to consent to the procedure.

Years ago "Doctor Knows Best" was a TV show. Now there is patient autonomy. The field has gone from only the health professional making the decision to letting the patient decide. The *Patient's Bill of Rights* gives the patient the right to decide and the right to refuse treatment even if fatal. Legally health professionals must obtain informed consent and cannot perform a potentially dangerous procedure without a patient's permission. If a patient is incompetent, then proxy consent is required. Yet patients who are sick enough to be hospitalized may or may not be competent enough to make such decisions. It is asking a lot to expect a patient to decide. Understanding is assumed after a patient says "I have no questions." The health professional often expects patients to comprehend statistics. Recommendations may be made, for example, regarding surgery vs. medication and the percent of the patient's risk with each procedure.

Most people, when their lives are threatened, just want help. When Informed Consent is requested, the patient may be experiencing fear, stress, unfamiliar surroundings, effects of pathology, and effects of treatment. Health professionals often subtly guide patients. They should, however, stimulate the patient to think through the decision.

It is important to (1) explain the better treatment reasoning (2) address the patient's need to know (3) enhance the patient's autonomy (4) enhance patients' control of their lives.

Often it is a matter of a value choice as in a cancer patient's choice of taking experimental drugs for six months or going home. There is no objectively right answer. In the end if the cancer patient wants to go home and go untreated, even though there is a chance of remission (getting better) with treatment, the patient should be allowed to do so.

The health care provider should:

1. understand that most patients are diminished in their ability to comprehend
2. be factual and supportive in short-term contact
3. avoid an assembly line approach although staff time is precious and scarce
4. reject the opportunity to decide for the patient; first tell the patient the options
5. determine what the patient actually understands
6. include a suggestion for the inefficient solution even though it takes more time

The occupational therapy assistant might be involved in dealing with a patient who must make important health care decisions or who is being asked to participate in an occupational therapy study. The occupational therapy assistant might be the health team member giving the information in order to obtain consent. The Occupational Therapy Code of Ethics includes informing those served of the nature and potential outcomes of occupational therapy services.

CODES OF PROFESSIONAL ETHICS

Professional obligations have been a part of ethical codes since the Hippocratic Oath. Yet, only recently have codes recognized patient's rights as well. Several associations have recently revised their codes. In some cases sections discouraging members from advertising were modified as a result of court decisions regarding restricted economic competition. Other revisions reflect a wider scope or condensations for clarity and enforceability.

The American Physical Therapy Association omitted loyalty to the profession from its 1981 revisions indicating that ethicists had criticized such codes as instruments for self preservation. Kirkwood Community College includes such a theme in its *Creed for COTAs* which follows. The American Dietetic Association added an enforcement process to its 1984 code. Most organizations state that the code is meant to guide the professional. The American Occupational Therapy Association's 1988 change includes a wide range of areas covering not only principles related to those serviced but to other health professionals and society as a whole. The preamble states that the term occupational therapist in the document includes registered occupational therapists, occupational therapy assistants, and occupational therapy students.

The length of the documents vary considerably with some organizations providing both a shorter list of standards and a longer guide for conduct. Titles or categories differ as well, however, content is of key importance. Although confidentiality is included in all codes, the approach of the overall documents can be very different. The primary focus of the 1980 American Medical Association (AMA) *Principles of Medical Ethics* is the physician's duty to benefit the patient. While the 1976 code of the American Nurses' Association (ANA) began by affirming the "self determination of clients." The AMA principles affirmed the right of each physician to choose the patients to be served (except in emergency) while the ANA code speaks of the right to quality health care for all. The occupational therapy (AOTA) document covers 6 principles related to autonomy/beneficence, competence, compliance with laws and regulations, public information, professional relationships, and professional conduct.

While codes of ethics provide standards and guidelines, enforcement is a separate issue. Katherine Reed, Chair of the AOTA Standards and Ethics Commission,[37] points out that "The AOTA ethics are a set of desired behaviors," that alleged violations of ethics should first be referred to the State licensure board (if the state has OT licensure), and that "the ultimate sanction that the

AOTA can apply is withdrawal of certification...only upon sound evidence of failure or unwillingness to follow the desired behavior." Areas of misconduct covered by State boards are in Table 16-1.

A related legal issue is that of malpractice. The American Occupational Therapy Association encourages both students and practitioners to carry individual liability insurance even though they may be working in a health care institution. Thomas Steich[38] states "Occupational therapists are responsible for their own actions, even though they may be following orders or employed by a health care facility. Occupational therapy personnel should follow safe and accepted practices and procedures, with the knowledge of the profession, and exercise reasonable judgement." Malpractice insurance rates for occupational therapy are relatively low, and occupational therapy assistant educational programs generally provide forms and processing for students as a group.

State licensing divisions print documents related to professional misconduct (Table 16-1) and often include them in copies of an Occupational Therapy Practice Act. Some state licensure boards will also research an area of concern and provide guidelines. In 1985 New York State issued practice guidelines which were the result of meetings of a Joint Practice Committee of the State Board for Occupational Therapy and the State Board for Physical Therapy.

An example of a therapeutic approach used in both occupational and physical therapy is shown in Figure 16-1. Moving the arm of a patient who does not have active muscle power, through its full range of motion keeps the joints from losing mobility and may promote return of muscle strength in an early stage of treatment. This will in turn help the patient to carry out daily living tasks.

This type of therapeutic approach requires the occupational therapy assistant to be skilled and knowledgeable and to use judgement in consultation with the supervising occupational therapist. Ethical considerations involve recognition of one's own abilities and limitations as well as being aware of guidelines regarding overlapping areas of practice with other licensed professions.

CREED FOR COTA'S[36]

As a Certified Occupational Therapy Assistant I have a responsibility to the professional group to which I belong, the institution to which I am attached and the community in which I live. This responsibility requires that I act and speak in such a manner that occupational therapy is presented favorably to the institution and the community, and the institution is presented favorably in the community. This requires that I maintain consistently high standards of performance as a therapeutically oriented person, that I respect channels of authority and am mindful that, if I criticize to outsiders that to which I belong, I degrade myself, whether it is the Association, occupational therapy, the institution or the department.

The American Occupational Therapy Association will provide me with general standards of performance, and a registered occupational therapist will provide me with supervision in my work. The welfare of the patient will at all times be uppermost in my mind. His dignity as a person will not permit me to be disrespectful of his person by 1) discussing him with anyone except authorized people, 2) mistreatment physically or mentally, or 3) assuming responsibility for his treatment above that consistent with my training and experience. To help maintain these standards, I will support my state and national organizations with dues and my service.

IN THE WORDS OF AN OCCUPATIONAL THERAPY ASSISTANT

I believe that when you feel positive about yourself, you cannot help but achieve more and perform better in your daily life activities. Since the origins of occupational therapy lie in restoring and maintaining functions in the individual client it is only natural for us to develop mind and body together.

The physically disabled person needs to develop a more realistic positive self concept in a world designed primarily for the able. Our clients benefited greatly from our therapies, but they let us know that they also needed someone to talk to. They had problems fitting into "normal" social situations, and wanted to know how to resolve some of these needs. Problems they wanted help with were, for example, how to deal with parents who still viewed them as children, and how and when to speak appropriately in a group social setting.

In our society, the disabled have been viewed negatively because of a lack of knowledge and understanding of their problems by the non-disabled. But now, through the formation of my psycho-social group our clients are encouraged to explore their own self-awareness and self concept as well as to work on skills to give them the ability to cope with confronting life situations.

Established by myself and a consulting OT, as one aspect of the group's plans, we encouraged everyone to begin keeping a journal. The journal was to become their daily form of communicating to themselves. In the journal they were to describe their self-improvement hopes, future plans, problem solving possibilities, and to identify feelings. During our meetings, some have chosen to share what they have written; others have not. The choice is theirs.[39]

Joanne Copley, COTA, BS
Adult Day Treatment Center
United Cerebral Palsy Center
Buffalo, New York

SUGGESTIONS

1. Review the principles covered in the *Occupational Therapy Code of Ethics* and identify the sections that are particularly important to you.
2. Begin to practice ethical principles in your daily activities and in your contacts with others.
3. Write to your State Licensure Board for a copy of the document dealing with professional misconduct.
4. Compare the code for occupational therapy with that for another health career.
5. Relate a recent medical ethics current event to an issue covered in a code of ethics.

READING OBJECTIVES

Autonomy

1. Define what is meant by a person (the concept of personhood)
   a) as stated by a philosopher
   b) in your own words
2. Name and discuss one fundamental moral principle which affects bioethical decisions.
3. State opinions as to whether the concept of autonomy differs for the infant, the institutionalized, the aged.
4. Identify ways in which autonomy affects the relationship between the health professional and the patient or client.
5. Give an example of patient autonomy in relation to the patient's family.

Medical Experimentation and Allocation of Scarce Resources

1. Give two examples of recent technological developments and a positive and negative reflection about each.
2. Explain what is meant by "scarce resources in health care."
3. List ways in which the allocation of scarce resources may be decided.
   a) Give two examples of ways in which scarce resources are currently allocated in health care institutions in the U.S.
   b) Discuss how you feel allocation should be handled.

Life/Death Considerations

1. Define euthanasia and its implications for OT students.
2. Give an example of how occupational therapy intervention could enable a child, who the parents might consider "better off dead," to function more productively.

3. Reflect on how you might motivate an older adult who says "Leave me alone, I'm ready to die."
4. Think about an occupational therapy strategy which might prove helpful for a dying patient.

Truth Telling and Confidentiality

1. Name the most long standing and universal ethical code inclusion for health professionals.
2. State the exceptional circumstances under which confidentiality may be violated.
3. Give an example as to how truth telling, lying and secrecy relate to the occupational therapy assistant.
4. Give reasons why a terminal diagnosis should or should not be revealed to a patient.

Informed Consent

1. Explain the meaning of informed consent.
2. Give examples of situations in which informed consent is important.
3. Reflect on whether or not you would share your feelings with a patient, your supervisor or the physician if you felt a patient should not consent to a particular treatment because of the risk-benefit ratio, or thought that occupational therapy techniques might provide some benefit with less risk.
4. Plan how an occupational therapy assistant would provide information about occupational therapy treatment to a patient so that the patient would fully understand and willingly participate.

Codes of Professional Ethics

1. Identify how codes of ethics may differ.
2. Name the issue included in virtually all codes of ethics in the health field.
3. Reflect on which of the Principles of Occupational Therapy Ethics might be hardest to follow.

REFERENCES

[32]Basson M: Ethics Humanism and Medicine. New York, Liss, 1980.

[33]Bak S: Lying-Word Choice in Public and Private Life. Pantheon, 1982.

[34]Beauchamp W: Bioethics. Wadsworth, 1982.

[35]Gorovitz: Moral Problems in Medicine. Prentiss Hall, 1983.

[36]Developed by Frank Lydic, Kirkwood Community College, Cedar Rapids, Iowa.

[37]Reed K: The Functions of Professional Ethics. OT News, June 1985.

[38]Steich T: Malpractice and Occupational Therapy Personnel. OT News, June 1985.

[39]Adapted from Development of a Psycho-Social Group for the Chronic Physically Disabled Adult. Advance, Vol. 2 No. 4, February 1986.

TABLE 16-1
ABUSES SUBJECT TO PENALTIES BY A STATE DIVISION OF PROFESSIONAL MISCONDUCT

Practice by an unlicensed person
Fraudulent or deceitful practice by licensed individuals
Practice beyond the authorized scope of the profession
Gross negligence or gross incompetence
Refusal to provide professional service on the basis of a client's racial, religious, or national background
Practice of the profession while the ability to practice is impaired by alcohol, narcotics, or by a physical or mental disability
Evidence that an applicant for licensure is of questionable moral character or is unfit to practice

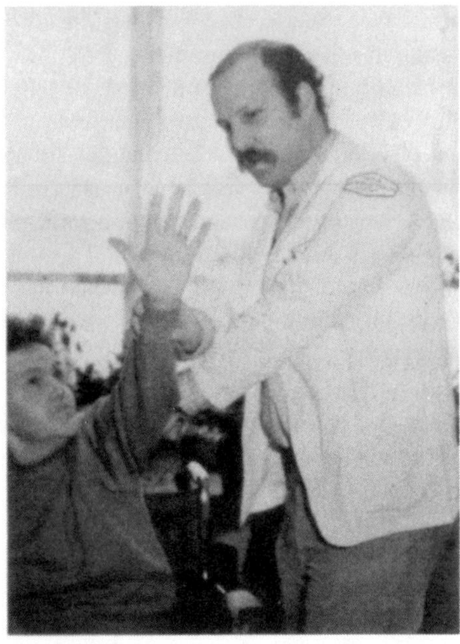

Figure 16-1: A skilled occupational therapy assistant assists a patient in moving her arm through its full range of motion.

CHAPTER 17

PROFESSIONAL INVOLVEMENT

GETTING INVOLVED PROFESSIONALLY

Being an occupational therapy assistant may be considered "just a job" or as an exciting opportunity to be part of a whole profession. The chapters in this book on professional organizations and on continuing education touched on areas for involvement. This chapter will further expand on such opportunities and offer actual examples of ways in which occupational therapy assistants contribute to the profession.

Most professional organizations offer the vital programs they do because of voluntary membership efforts. Those local OT individuals who plan, carry out and evaluate conferences are volunteers. Those speaking generally do so without payment. Those serving on an editorial committee of a professional publication, writing a book review or publishing an article are generally not paid. Officers of an organization, committee members and other members who offer and provide temporary efforts to promote the objectives of the organization do not expect any monetary gain.

Reasons for Participation

Why get involved one might ask. The benefits are many. "Occupational therapy" is a key one. Each of us can benefit from being occupied in purposeful activity. Some of the goals that may sound familiar as appropriate for the recipients of the services of an occupational therapy assistant may be important for the occupational therapy assistant as well. Increased socialization, better self image, sense of responsibility, improved skills, diversion from concerns which cannot be changed, self identity, enhanced communication, socially acceptable relating and others are all possible.

One of the most significant reasons for professional involvement is recognition within the field. This happens as the person and the person's name become known within the profession. Recognition may be specifically expressed via an award or written acknowledgement but more often it comes as the individual begins to be sought out as a speaker, author, as co-worker on a project, or for advice in an area of expertise. Such an individual creates a stimulating reaction when entering a professional group or draws an audience when announced as attending a meeting. And of course, the benefits with regard to job opportunities are many. Professional involvement listed on a resume may often be the reason one equally qualified candidate will be chosen for a job over another. An employer may also seek out a recognized occupational therapy assistant and offer a position before it is even announced.

Sometimes beginning occupational therapy assistants or students are in awe of a recognized individual within the field and believe it is not possible for them to achieve such status. But each of those recognized individuals started out by just getting involved. Making a commitment to a particular task or goal perhaps in a specialty area, is one way. Letting people know about what you've done (perhaps through a presentation or article) is another. But just making yourself available to occupational therapy organizations wherever needed is equally important and allows you to develop your own sense of direction as you learn about the field and how the organization operates.

A major reason for participation is to promote occupational therapy. If you believe in its benefits, why not let others find out about it?

Ways to Promote Occupational Therapy

How to get involved is an easier matter once you've made the decision to do so. Many approaches mean just being a good citizen.

Write your legislative representative when there's an issue you wish to support or oppose. Professional newsletters usually identify legislative proposals and their progress through the system. Requests for support or opposition of a proposed bill are sent to occupational therapy program directors who in turn alert their students to the need to write letters. An example of such a request was for support of occupational therapy as a Medicare inclusion. The volume of letters is monitored by congressional representatives, senators, and state representatives. A volume of such letters often assures passage of legislation for State licensure or practice acts.

Write a letter to the editor of your favorite paper about occupational therapy or an issue related to it. When occupational therapy was mentioned on a TV soap opera, there were many letters in general newspapers which were both in favor of it because of the publicity and against it because of the way the term was used. Professional publications also publish letters to the editor. The "American Journal of Occupational Therapy" ran letters for several months on the question as to whether the journal cover should have a picture or just the list of topics covered in the issue.

The "COTA Share" column in *Occupational Therapy News* presented a marvelous opportunity for occupational therapy assistants and students to share their views and their expertise. Contributions on issues of a general nature as well as specifically relevant to the COTA are now being included in *OT Week*.

High school career days represent a marvelous chance to return to your former school or neighborhood to speak about your new career choice or explorations, to test out your ideas about a potential career, compare it to others, and ask questions or receive literature from other representatives in the field. Staffing a table at a career fair provides an opportunity to sell yourself on OT as you answer questions for others. You'll usually find yourself emphasizing the positive aspects of being an occupational therapy assistant.

Open house programs at hospitals also provide an opportunity for give and take in terms of asking and answering questions and observing or demonstrating occupational therapy techniques. These programs are often scheduled in conjunction with special occasions such as the anniversary of the health care facility or Health Promotion Week.

Occupational Therapy Week celebrations are a fun time to try out unique ideas and get publicity for them. In addition to National Occupational Therapy Week which is usually the week of the American Occupational Therapy Association Annual Conference, there are also state and city occupational therapy weeks proclaimed. The American Student Committee of the Occupational Therapy Association (ASCOTA) Reference Handbook suggests that students plan for Occupational Therapy Week well in advance and perhaps even select and celebrate a week which is most convenient for the group. Suggestions include holding an open house or party, placing a series of radio and television public service announcements, setting up a bulletin board with photos of current practice and or old photos of occupational therapy in the past, making a display of adaptive equipment or activities for use in local public libraries or college libraries, having National Occupational Therapy Week recognized on marquees or display boards in the community, honoring an occupational therapy assistant with a ceremony, providing entertainment at a nursing home, providing display posters for buses, sending suggestions for feature articles to feature editors of newspapers and magazines, or offering a list of suggested occupational therapy assistant guests and topics for presentation to a radio or television talk show host or producer. Among the special events suggested are an art show or sports event where disabled people can demonstrate their independence, a rehabilitation fair demonstrating services and equipment, community health education seminars, or a health fair.[40]

Public displays as shown in preparation in Figure 17-1, involve the OTA for both professional and therapeutic purposes. Activities might include promoting Occupational Therapy Week, career day or "Open House" to inform the public about occupational therapy, arranging a display to show patients and families helpful equipment, or a fair or sale to demonstrate or sell projects actually made by clients. Patients may be involved directly in preparing posters, arranging the display or actually explaining or demonstrating an activity to visitors, all of which helps patients achieve such therapeutic goals as taking responsibility, gaining self esteem, working with others, and developing skills towards being organized.

The 'OT Line is the name of the newsletter of the American Student Committee of the Occupational Therapy Association (ASCOTA). It is interested in receiving any type of news from occupational therapy or occupational therapy assistant students or just short items or letters about what's happening. *JOTS*, the *Journal of Occupational Therapy Students* welcomes longer articles.

OT Student Clubs exist at many occupational therapy assistant schools and provide an opportunity to get involved not only with occupational therapy but with the student government or student affairs office at the college. The clubs generally elect officers and hold meetings or functions at regular intervals. Programs might feature speakers and be open to all students at the college.

ASCOTA or the American Student Committee of the Occupational Therapy Association which is described in the chapter on professional organizations provides an opportunity for occupational therapy assistant students to get involved on a national level. Occupational therapy assistant students who served as ASCOTA officers, usually as OTA Vice Chair, have later continued their involvement. Some have become officers in other areas of the American Occupational Therapy Association (AOTA) and continued their participation in occupational therapy activities after graduation. To run for office students should submit basic biographical information and an essay describing why they are particularly appropriate for the position. The nominating committee selects two students for each office, then all student members vote by mail.

State and local occupational therapy associations offer many opportunities for occupational therapy assistant and student involvement. Many such organizations have a COTA liaison position. There are opportunities to serve on committees or as a chairperson. Specialty sections provide for presentations and discussions on topics of interest. There may be special student meetings as well as general membership and business meetings. Public relations is an important area for participation as is assisting in preparing and distributing a newsletter. Even the job placement announcements need to be coordinated, and the person who works on them is the first to know about new job openings. Many State associations name a COTA of the Year.

AOTA or the American Occupational Therapy Association recognizes occupational therapy assistants via two major honors: the Award of Excellence; and the Roster of Honor which entitles recipients to use the initials ROH after their names. These awards are granted to individuals who have participated actively and extensively on a national level. Opportunities for participation include the Recognition or Certification Committees, the Commission on Practice (on which the ASCOTA OTA Vice Chair serves) or the Commission on

Education where COTAs may serve as the fieldwork representative from an educational program. The major form of participation for COTAs is at annual conferences where they might present papers, help plan and make the conference run smoothly, sell OT items to support a particular project, visit or operate an exhibit, design a display, meet and greet other COTAs, and, of course, attend sessions. In 1989 there were celebrations of the 30th anniversary of the COTA at both the AOTA annual conference and state and regional events.

PUBLICATIONS AND PRESENTATIONS

In recent years occupational therapy assistants have increasingly published and presented papers at professional meetings. This has been encouraged through special opportunities such as regional COTA meetings, COTA Forums at professional conferences and the "COTA Share" column in "Occupational Therapy News," the newspaper of the American Occupational Therapy Association. Many COTAs have collaborated with OTRs and other professionals on articles for professional journals such as "The American Journal of Occupational Therapy" as well as for textbooks and other publications.

Examples of published writings and of professional presentation by COTAs are included in this chapter. The range of topics is quite broad. COTAs have written on subjects as diverse as their feelings about the profession to occupational therapy treatment techniques or research.

Table 17-1 gives examples of COTA Forum presentations at AOTA conferences. Table 17-2 is a bibliographical listing of selected works by COTAs. And Table 17-3 lists representative papers presented by COTAs.

Perhaps the simplest way an occupational therapy assistant can get in print and at the same time learn and help others to learn is by submitting a topic of interest to "Member Hotline" a column in "Occupational Therapy News." The column offers a way to communicate with the entire membership when seeking or offering information. It usually focuses on treatment areas and thus serves to inform the OTA of new areas of practice. The table which lists sample topics submitted by COTAs is included in the chapter on the occupational therapy assistant.

The 'OT Line encourages students to submit articles on any topic.

IN THE WORDS OF AN OCCUPATIONAL THERAPY ASSISTANT

The first critical responsibility is involvement in our professional organizations. I am well aware of the anticipated dread of becoming an executive board

member. But that's where the action is. Volunteer for COTA representative for your district; run for office; edit the newsletter. Do something! How about writing a "Practice Paper" to share your ideas with your fellow colleagues at your district or state conference? Have you ever thought about writing an article for a magazine, your local newspaper or for other professional journals? This can be very creative and rewarding. Under the AOTA reorganizational plan, a COTA can represent a region in the Representative Assembly. How about it?[41]
Terry D. Brittell, COTA, ROH
Member COTA Task Force

SUGGESTIONS

1. Try one or more of the ideas for getting involved.
2. Read an article written by an occupational therapy assistant.
3. Attend a presentation by an occupational therapy assistant
4. Participate in a career day or OT Open House.
5. Watch for Occupational Therapy Week announcements.

READING OBJECTIVES

1. List approaches for professional involvement.
2. Identify the two national honors available for COTAs.
3. Give examples of the topics of publications and presentations by occupational therapy assistants.
4. Name the column in "Occupational Therapy News" through which COTAs can request information on topics of interest.
5. State the procedure for becoming an officer in ASCOTA and the benefits of professional involvement.

REFERENCES

[40]ASCOTA Reference Handbook, American Occupational Therapy Association, Initiated 1982.

[41]Excerpted from Mental Health Specialty Section Newsletter, a publication of the American Occupational Therapy Association, Vol. 3, No. 3, 1980.

TABLE 17-1
EXAMPLES OF COTA FORUM PRESENTATIONS BY COTAs

Awareness Group
A Handful of Opportunity through a Work Activity Program
A COTA Initiated Program for Visually Handicapped Patients
COTA as Department Head
Enrichment for the Regressed Geriatric Resident
Playing the Guitar with One Hand and One Foot
Group Dynamics with the Elderly
Clowning as a Therapeutic Approach
Developing a Day Program for the Adult Developmentally Disabled
Historical Background of the COTA
Effective OTR/COTA Relationships Through a Co-Treatment Model
Video Games: Therapeutic Implications for Patient Training and Recreation
COTA and OTR Collaboration in Student Supervision

TABLE 17-2
EXAMPLES OF THE VARIETY OF PUBLICATIONS BY COTAs

Black, Wendy, et al: Development of a Hand Sensitivity Test for the Hypersensitive Hand. American Journal of Occupational Therapy, Vol. 37, No. 3, 1983.
Brittell, Terry D: Ramifications of a COTA Title Change. Occupational Therapy News, February 1987.
Brittell, Terry D: The Transition from Institution to Community. Occupational Therapy in the Community, 1977 NYSOT Association.
Coffey, Peggy: OTA Education. Education Bulletin, AOTA, March 1986.
Copley, Joanne: Development of a Psycho-Social Group for the Chronic Physically Disabled Adult. Advance: A Weekly News Exchange for Occupational Therapists, February 1986.
Cox, Betty, et al: How to Apply for a Job on Paper...and Get the Interview. American Occupational Therapy Association, 1977.
Curley, Joleen: Leading Poetry Writing Groups in a Nursing Home Activities Program. Physical & Occupational Therapy in Geriatrics, 1982.
Higbie, Carlynn: Low Birthweight Infants: Early Intervention and Stimulation Programs. Journal of Occupational Therapy Students, 1986.
Klausner, Bracha: Spling. United States Patent Office Trademark, 1974.
Knapp, Ruth: Book Review of An Easier Way: Handbook for the Elderly and Handicapped. American Journal of Occupational Therapy, 1983.
Nardiello-Erickson, Josephine: Occupational Therapy Protocol Book for Designated Activities on an Intensive Treatment Therapy Unit. Bronx Psychiatric Center, 1982.
Pinto, Gertrude: The COTAs Book of Crafts. Publication forthcoming.
Rehmeyer, Nancy: "COTAs in Baltimore County Public Schools." Developmental Disabilities: Special Interest Section Newsletter, Vol. 2, No. 2, 1979.
Ryan, Sally: The Certified Occupational Therapy Assistant: Roles and Responsibilities. Slack Inc., 1986.

TABLE 17-3
EXAMPLES OF PROFESSIONAL PRESENTATIONS BY OCCUPATIONAL THERAPY ASSISTANTS

Amble, Debora: Body Mechanics Workshop. Auburn, Washington Conference, 1979.

Barlton, Sherry: Role of Volunteer Coordinator in Nursing Homes. Tri-State Hospital Assembly Conference, 1973.

Barlton, Sherry: Occupational Therapy with the Client with Obesity. North Dakota OTA Annual Conference, 1975.

Brittell, Terry: Stress Management Workshop. Hospital Presentations.

Brown, Ilenna: Free to Be...Elimination of Architectural and Emotional Barriers. New Providence Board of Education, 1978.

Brown, Pamela: The Role of an Occupational Therapy Assistant. California Occupational Therapy Association Conference, 1981.

Ciampa, Marcella, D'Errico, Linda, Kornick, Susan, Mallard, Joyce: Role of COTAs in the Hospital Setting. Northeast Region Student Conference, 1982.

Cox, Betty: Advocacy in Action. Wisconsin Occupational Therapy Association Annual Conference, 1981.

Dlugos, Tom: COTA in Unique Role (Orthotics). NYSOTA Conference, 1974.

Freeman, Michelle: COTA Role. Alabama COTA Conference, 1983.

Hewlett, Bernice: Homemaking in a Therapeutic Environment. New York State Occupational Therapy Conference, 1974.

Hipson, Regina: Benefits of COTAs and OTRs Working Together to Meet Patients' Needs. Massachusetts OT Association Annual Meeting, 1982.

Johnson, Shirley: Occupational Therapy Visibility in Mental Health. Ohio Occupational Therapy Assistants Conference, May 1984.

Kramer, Lorraine, Peralta, Angela, Pinto, Gertrude: New Roles for COTAs in OT Educational Settings. Northeast Student Conference, 1982.

Lopez, Nancy: Award Winning Paper. Great Southern OT Conference, 1983.

Sarabia, Alice: Physical Medicine in a State Hospital. NYSOTA Conference, 1984.

Seltser, Charlotte: Personal Experiences, Ideas and Guidelines for Working with the Visually Impaired. Southeast COTA Conference, 1981.

Springer, Truman: Marketing Your OT Device. First NYS COTA Conference, May 1987.

Tumiel, John: Career Alternatives for COTAs. Southeast COTA Conference, 1981.

Volenda, Beth Ann, Giangrosso, Joann, Mason, Susan, Salter, Terry: Treatment Approaches with CVA Patients. Southeast COTA Conference, 1981.

Wolcott, Rose: The Computer as a Therapeutic Tool. American Occupational Therapy Association Conference, 1984.

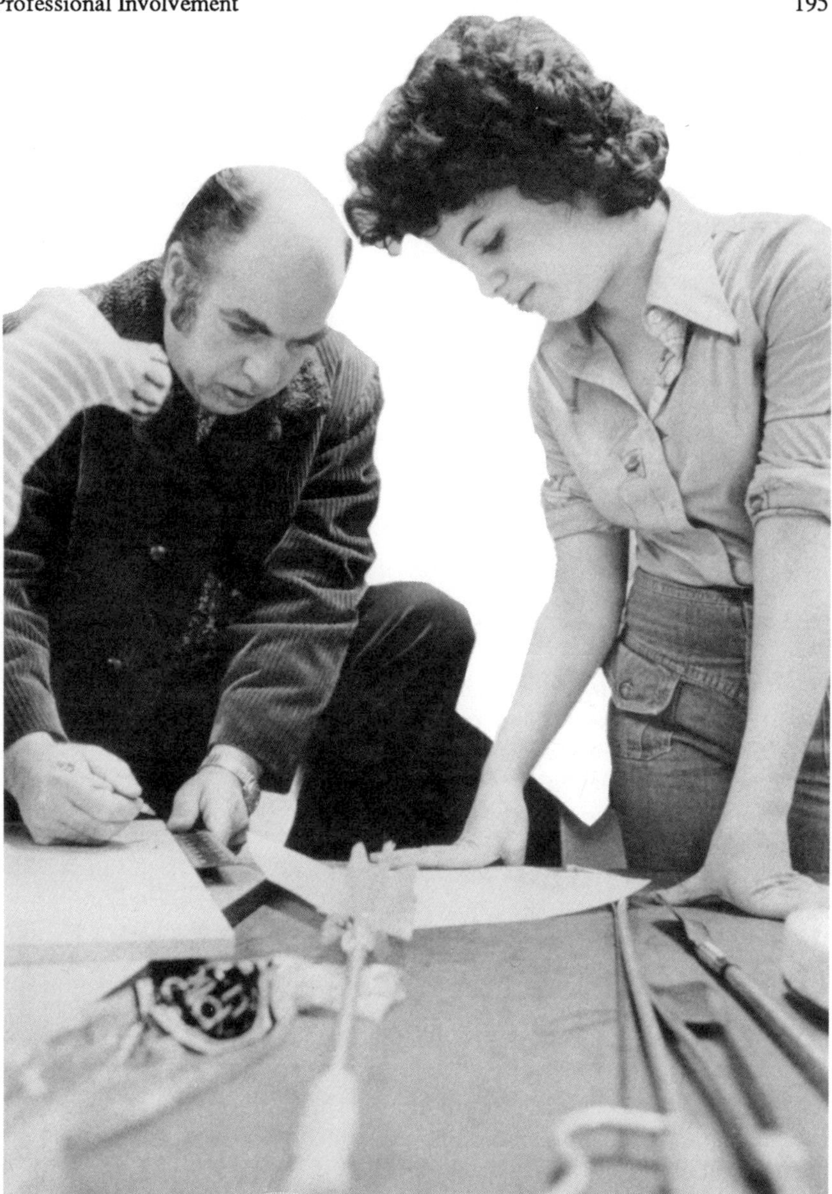

Figure 17-1: Assistive devices such as a long handled brush, reacher and shoehorn can often help an individual to be independent in self care. The occupational therapy assistant student shown gets help in preparing a display showing the benefits of such devices and their use in occupational therapy.

CHAPTER 18

FUTURE TRENDS

INTRODUCTION

Occupational therapy is a growing field. The occupational therapy assistant is becoming increasingly recognized as an important member of the health care team. Changes in the health care delivery system are reflected in the field of occupational therapy as well.

PRACTICE

In the realm of practice there is an increasing trend toward shorter hospital stays. Community based care is receiving an increasing emphasis by occupational therapists. Occupational therapy assistants are continuing to treat the aged as the national population's average age continues to rise, but they are also increasingly being recruited for work with the population under age 20. This is particularly true for the developmentally disabled and in the school systems as a result of legislative efforts to recognize "handicapped" children and provide them with services to maximize their potential.

Examples of new roles for COTAs were presented in Chapter 11. The concept of occupational therapy assistants working in occupational therapy educational programs was new when proposed in 1973. By 1985 30% of the programs had COTA faculty. Rehabilitation supply companies are increasingly seeking occupational therapy personnel. The increase in cancer survival rates is leading to more occupational therapy personnel in both cancer rehabilitation and in hospice care. Although many school districts have not yet established specific titled positions for the occupational therapy assistant, OTAs are being hired increasingly in such settings as teaching assistants, therapy assistants or through outside agencies which rotate occupational therapy assistants through schools. The job lines can be expected to follow.

Occupational therapy is being recognized as important in many areas of need. There are occupational therapy assistants working in obesity and in stress reduction programs for both clients and health care staff.

The increasing developments in prevention and treatment techniques in health care are expected to affect the kinds of patients treated by occupational therapy assistants. Patients with disabilities such as hemiplegia resulting from strokes currently constitute the largest single category of diagnoses treated by occupational therapy assistants. This is expected to decrease as are patients with complications following heart attacks. While at the same time early recognition of cancer and approaches which prolong life thereafter will likely lead to increasing numbers of patients with residual effects of cancer being treated in occupational therapy.

The health care delivery system is experiencing remarkable changes in financing and marketing of services. Treatment is increasingly being provided by the private sector rather than in government institutions. Humana Hospital, known for its pioneering efforts in artificial heart transplants, is an example of the type of for-profit health care institution that could be expected to employ greater numbers of occupational therapy personnel in the future. In keeping with the increasing emphasis on cost effectiveness more health care programs are beginning to offer occupational therapy services on weekends and in the evenings as well as the traditional 9–5 hours. This trend may increase with the requirement by the federal government of Prospective Payment and Diagnostic Related Groups (DRGs). Under this system health care providers can expect to receive a set sum of money based on an estimated pre-set number of days (average length of stay) of treatment anticipated on a national basis by diagnosis. Thus it is to the hospital's advantage to provide all the necessary treatments including occupational therapy in as short a time as possible as the hospital will be reimbursed for average days of treatment, for example, for a Medicare stroke patient whether the patient remains 10 days or 25 days. Thus occupational therapy personnel may no longer have the luxury of the patient remaining in the institution while, for example, awaiting an assistive device which will enable the patient to function more independently upon discharge. More intensive treatment may result with a variety of occupational therapy goals being approached simultaneously, perhaps after the evening meal as well as during the traditional daytime hours. With the expected earlier discharge of such patients, occupational therapy personnel will be needed to provide extended treatment once the patient returns to the community. This trend toward shorter hospital stays and increased community based therapy services is appearing in mental health services (deinstitutionalization) as well as in general medical care. OT goals are being written as measurable outcomes more frequently to justify reimbursement under new government guidelines.

The American Occupational Therapy Association identified eight changes expected into the early 1990s which should increase the requirements for occupational therapy manpower.[14] These are listed in Table 18-1. James

Garibaldi[42] in commenting on John Naisbitt's (Megatrends) projections reflected "The practice of occupational therapy calls for a great deal of innovation and initiative and fosters a spirit of entrepreneurship...Mr. Naisbitt's projections for the future bode well for occupational therapy as health care and fitness assumes its position as a primary economic growth area."

EDUCATION

The trend in education of the occupational therapy assistant in the United States is clearly toward training at the Associate degree level. The American Occupational Therapy Association in its 1983 Essentials for an Occupational Therapy Assistant Training Program[18] introduced the requirement that training be provided in conjunction with an institution of higher education. This insures that even in certificate programs the education obtained will be acceptable toward continued education toward a degree.

The occupational therapy profession is continually studying the educational requirements for entry to the profession. Under consideration was mandating an associate degree for the occupational therapy assistant and a master's degree for the occupational therapist. Currently the occupational therapy assistant can enter the field by completing an approved program at either a certificate level or an associate degree level. And the occupational therapist can enter the field by completing an accredited program at either a baccalaureate degree or master's degree level. If the master's degree become the entry point there would be a greater difference in the educational preparation between the occupational therapy assistant and the occupational therapist. The American Occupational Therapy Association committee recommended no change at present.

The list of approved technical education programs (Appendix) continues to identify programs which offer a certificate program, but the list of developing programs are primarily at the associate degree level. In 1988, 62 programs offered associate degrees while only 6 continued to offer certificate programs.

The American Occupational Therapy Association has been responsive to trends affecting the profession and as a result has changed educational requirements accordingly. In its April 1985 document, *Occupational Therapy Manpower: A Plan for Progress*, suggestions related to education include: updating the Essentials to allow for fieldwork in more "non-traditional" settings including home health agencies, free-standing outpatient centers, private industry, and adult day care centers; encouraging the occupational therapy educational system to ensure that entry-level graduates are equipped with knowledge and skills in marketing, health economics, systems behavior and networking, management, clinical reporting systems, and application of computer technology for clinical management and patient treatment and evaluation; updating the role delineation to add emphasis on contracted services, long-term care, hospice, health promotion/wellness, and industrial/occupational health; developing educational resources to increase practitioner's skills in clinical areas which include cancer rehabilitation, gerontology/long-term care, health promotion/wellness, health screening, home health, retirement planning and stress management; encouraging the development of "non-traditional" programs to serve populations such as second career seekers which might include part-time programs, weekend and evening programs, independent study programs, work-study programs, concentrated short-term programs, and life experience credit programs.

PERSONNEL

The registered occupational therapist and the certified occupational therapy assistant will continue to be the two credentialed categories of personnel in the field of occupational therapy although the occupational therapy aide is often included as a third category of OT personnel. Areas of greatest shortage of COTAs are in the Southeast and in the West. Since it has been shown that COTAs tend to practice in the states in which they have been trained, encouragement of new educational programs in those areas is likely to result in increased personnel. Figure 18-1 shows the growth of COTAs by state.

There continues to be a demand for occupational therapy personnel which exceeds the supply. Patterns of employment often reflect changes in the health care system. Manpower demands are expected to increase in long-term care, in school systems, and in community based and home health programs.

The American Occupational Therapy Association projects growth in the profession based on an expectation of 800 occupational therapy assistant graduates per year and a gradual increase in the output of occupational therapy educational programs. It reports in "Occupational Therapy Manpower: A Plan for Progress" dated April 1985:

> The growth of occupational therapy manpower through the mid to late 1970s exceeded most other health professions, and in fact exceeded most other occupations of any kind. Part of that growth was the result of the overall expansion of the health care system, part was the result of a high level of federal funding support for allied health education, and part was the result of greater awareness of the value of rehabilitative services...the best possible situation for the profession would be to grow at a constant rate, ideally at the same rate as the growth in requirements.

The Association has suggested the need to direct recruitment strategies to increase minority representation in the profession and to target population such as second career seekers, underemployed persons in related fields, and other older populations.

STATE REGULATION

By 1989, 46 jurisdictions had occupational therapy regulatory laws. This trend has been increasing rapidly. Thirty five states plus the District of Columbia and Puerto Rico are licensed. The remainder have registration, certification or trademark laws. Most require successful completion of the national certification examination.

The American Occupational Therapy Association continues to be the only organization which certifies occupational therapy personnel. The association has engaged a testing agency, Assessment Systems Inc., to administer certification examinations. Scoring is based on a scale rather than an absolute number of correct questions. Test questions reflect the role delineation of the OTR and COTA. Since the roles of occupational therapy personnel are changing, a new role delineation is proposed for approval in 1990. The American Occupational Therapy Certification Board has been asked to consider approaches to enable foreign students to achieve a higher success rate on the certification examinations. Such approaches might include offering the exam in Spanish or allowing more time for those for whom English is a second language. Although there are an increasing number of educational programs for support level occupational therapy personnel in other countries, there is no World Federation of Occupational Therapists mechanism for approval of such programs, so foreign educated assistants are not directly eligible for the certification examination for COTAs at the present time.

THERAPEUTIC ACTIVITIES

Types of treatment modalities and approaches are also reflecting general trends. With increased technology new devices are appearing on the market geared toward specific forms of treatment and toward enabling the patient to have increasing independence in activities of daily living. Thus computers are appearing in occupational therapy departments not only to maintain data for quality assurance reports but to evaluate and train patients in such areas as perception, eye hand coordination, reaction time, and pre-vocational skills.

Beginning approaches to socialization often start with parallel play. Two individuals playing a computer game are aware of each other but don't have to have much interaction. The areas of electronics and robotics are expanding and the latter is particularly relevant in enabling the physically challenged to handle self care. Self care evaluation and training is a key function of the occupational therapy assistant. Feeding devices are already in use in occupational therapy departments which enable a person who cannot lift a spoon or direct it to the mouth to eat from one that scoops food and positions it electronically.

Related to this is the relatively new approach to using trained animals, particularly monkeys, to perform daily living tasks for the disabled, such as feeding or getting clothes from a closet. While older related approaches remain in use, newer ones provide additional options. Occupational therapy assistants still make built up handles for utensils so that someone with poor grasp can handle a spoon but at the same time, they can consider more elaborate solutions where necessary. Crafts remain an important therapeutic activity (Figure 18-1) even as other approaches are gaining attention. The term "pet therapy" is heard more frequently in occupational therapy as the value of animals for psychological and sociological benefits is increasingly being recognized. Occupational therapy programs, particularly in psychiatric facilities and in nursing homes, are utilizing this approach which involves the senses of touch, sight, sound and smell. Positive emotional responses and enhanced communication have resulted.

Although crafts are still valued as therapeutic activities, as governmental regulations increasingly require measurable outcomes, there is a trend toward greater emphasis on other therapeutic approaches such as self care. Thus, the activity promoted in Figure 18-1, a Craft Fair, is seen less frequently. Occupational therapy assistants are involved in preparing such public displays for both professional and therapeutic purposes.

The occupational therapy assistant can look forward to an exciting career, one that has a sound base but which allows for the excitement of introducing new approaches as they evolve.

IN THE WORDS OF AN OCCUPATIONAL THERAPY ASSISTANT

Due to increased emphasis on deinstitutionalization and the need for appropriate programming to facilitate these trends, staff sharing was established with Way Station, a psychosocial rehabilitation program. Although I am employed by a hospital center, I was trained one day a week for four months at Way Station to increase my knowledge of community based programming and to examine the appropriateness of hospital based programs. Way Station has three units, food, clerical and maintenance, and services 75 individuals with an average daily attendance of 35.

At the end of my training I knew that a COTA with knowledge, skills and experience assumes a meaningful and purposeful role in psychosocial programs. COTAs assist their members to make the transition from patient to private citizen. In addition, patient treatment programs for the chronic adult population must continue to focus on self care, basic living skills including cooking, health, safety and money management, use of public transportation and social interactions. All of these programs can be provided by a COTA.

Alice Arthur, COTA[42]
Way Station, Inc.
Frederick, MD

SUGGESTIONS

1. Read the American Occupational Therapy Association's publications regarding future trends.
2. Read the new technology column in *AJOT*.
3. Talk with occupational therapists and assistants with years of experience in the field about the trends they have observed in practice.
4. Think about how new types of technology and products on the market might be used therapeutically.
5. Be aware of news items covering issues such as government regulations affecting health care including DRGs or malpractice and licensure concerns. Consider the implications for occupational therapy.

READING OBJECTIVES

1. Identify two trends in the practice of occupational therapy and the reasons for them.
2. Recognize whether occupational therapy education is moving toward increased years of schooling or less training.
3. Give the areas of occupational therapy where more personnel are expected to be needed.
4. Compare the number of states with occupational therapy licensure and the future expectations.
5. Give examples of newer therapeutic activities being used by occupational therapists and assistants.

REFERENCES

[42]Garibaldi, James, Executive Director, AOTA; Occupational Therapy Newspaper, November 1984, Megatrends and Beyond.

[42]Adapted from "The Role of the COTA in a Psychosocial Program." Occupational Therapy News, September 1984.

TABLE 18-1
CHANGES IN HEALTH CARE EXPECTED TO INCREASE REQUIREMENTS FOR OCCUPATIONAL THERAPY PERSONNEL

More societal emphasis on health promotion/disease prevention as well as a similar push from large private industries will result in more wellness programs.

More treatment needs will develop among cancer patients as more survive with disabilities.

More school-based practitioners will be needed because of the short-term increase in the size of the school-aged population and the likely increase in numbers of handicapped children.

Increased patient dependency on technology or equipment (such as dialysis or respirators) will require more adaptation of restricted environments.

There will be an increase in health maintenance programs, particularly for the elderly, as well as more alternative residential arrangements, such as elderly day care.

The emergence of Social Health Maintenance Organizations (SHMOs) will provide opportunities for occupational therapy personnel as case managers and integrators of social/health care factors.

Advances in technology will result in more opportunities for independence among the elderly and severely disabled, and a greater survival rate of children with birth defects.

Greater emphasis on rehabilitation of head trauma will result in the emergence of more head trauma programs.

Source: Occupational Therapy Manpower: A Plan for Progress.[14] American Occupational Therapy Association, 1985.

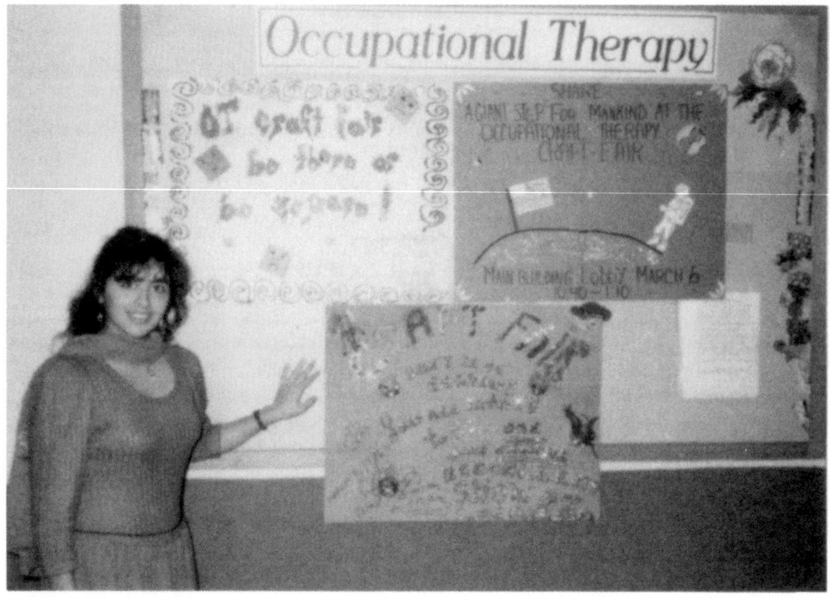

Figure 18-1: An occupational therapy assistant at a display designed to promote public awareness of the field.

APPENDICES

APPENDIX I

UNIFORM TERMINOLOGY FOR OCCUPATIONAL THERAPY—SECOND EDITION

Uniform Terminology—Second Edition may be used in a variety of ways. It defines occupational therapy practice, which includes **OCCUPATIONAL PERFORMANCE AREAS** and **OCCUPATIONAL PERFORMANCE COMPONENTS.**

Some examples of the differences between **OCCUPATIONAL PERFORMANCE AREAS** and **OCCUPATIONAL PERFORMANCE COMPONENTS** and programs and interventions are

1. An individual who is injured on the job may be able to return to work, which is an **OCCUPATIONAL PERFORMANCE AREA.** In order to achieve the outcome of returning to work, the individual may need to address specific **PERFORMANCE COMPONENTS** such as strength, endurance, and time management. The occupational therapist, in cooperation with the vocational team, utilizes planned interventions to achieve the desired outcome. These interventions may include activities such as an exercise program, body mechanics instruction, and job modification, and may be provided in a work-hardening program.
2. An individual with severe physical limitations may need and desire the opportunity to live within a community-integrated setting, which represents the **OCCUPATIONAL PERFORMANCE AREAS** of activities of daily living and work. In order to achieve the outcome of community living, the individual may need to address specific **PERFORMANCE COMPONENTS,** such as normalizing muscle tone, gross motor coordination, postural control, and self-management. The occupational therapist, in cooperation with the team, utilizes planned interventions to achieve the desired outcome. Interventions may include neuromuscular facilitation, object manipulation, instruction in use of adaptive equipment, use of environmental control systems, and functional positioning for eating. These interventions may be provided in a community-based independent living program.
3. A child with learning disabilities may need to perform educational activities within a public school setting. Since learning is a student's work, this educational activity would be considered the **OCCUPATIONAL PERFORMANCE AREA** for this individual. In order to achieve the educational outcome of efficient and effective completion of written classroom work, the child may need to address specific **OCCUPATIONAL PERFORMANCE COMPONENTS,** including sensory processing, perceptual skills, postural control, and motor skills. The occupational therapist, in cooperation with the team, utilizes planned interventions to achieve the desired outcome. Interventions may include activities such as adapting the student's seating to improve postural control and stability and practicing motor control and coordination. This program could be provided by school district personnel or through contracted services.
4. An infant with cerebral palsy may need to participate in developmental activities to engage in the **OCCUPATIONAL PERFORMANCE AREAS** of activities of daily living

and play. The developmental outcomes may be achieved by addressing specific **PERFORMANCE COMPONENTS** such as sensory awareness and neuromuscular control. The occupational therapist, in cooperation with the team, utilizes planned interventions to achieve the desired outcomes. Interventions may include activities such as seating and positioning for play, neuromuscular facilitation techniques to enable eating, and parent training. These interventions may be provided in a home-based occupational therapy program.

5. An adult with schizophrenia may need and desire to live independently in the community, which represents the **OCCUPATIONAL PERFORMANCE AREAS** of activities of daily living, work activities, and play or leisure activities. The specific **OCCUPATIONAL PERFORMANCE AREAS** may be medication routine, functional mobility, home management, vocational exploration, play or leisure performance, and social skills. In order to achieve the outcome of living alone, the individual may need to address specific **PERFORMANCE COMPONENTS** such as topographical orientation, memory, categorization, problem solving, interests, social conduct, and time management. The occupational therapist, in cooperation with the team, utilizes planned interventions to achieve the desired outcome. Interventions may include activities such as training in the use of public transportation, instruction in budgeting skills, selection of and participation in social activities, and instruction in social conduct. These interventions may be provided in a community-based mental health program.
6. An individual who abuses substances may need to reestablish family roles and responsibilities, which represents the **OCCUPATIONAL PERFORMANCE AREAS** of activities of daily living and work. In order to achieve the outcome of family participation, the individual may need to address the **PERFORMANCE COMPONENTS** of roles, values, social conduct, self-expression, coping skills, and self-control. The occupational therapist, in cooperation with the team, utilizes planned intervention to achieve the desired outcomes. Interventions may include role and value clarification exercises, role-playing, instruction in stress management techniques, and parenting skills. These interventions may be provided in an inpatient acute care unit.

OCCUPATIONAL THERAPY ASSESSMENT

Assessment is the planned process of obtaining, interpreting, and documenting the functional status of the individual.

OCCUPATIONAL THERAPY INTERVENTION

Occupational therapy addresses function and uses specific procedures and activities to (a) develop, maintain, improve, and/or restore the performance of necessary functions; (b) compensate for dysfunction; (c) minimize or prevent debilitation; and/or (d) promote health and wellness.

I. OCCUPATIONAL PERFORMANCE AREAS

A. Activities of Daily Living

1. *Grooming*—Obtain and use supplies to shave; apply and remove cosmetics; wash, comb, style, and brush hair; care for nails; care for skin; and apply deodorant.
2. *Oral Hygiene*—Obtain and use supplies; clean mouth and teeth; remove, clean, and reinsert dentures.
3. *Bathing*—Obtain and use supplies; soap, rinse, and dry all body parts; maintain bathing position; transfer to and from bathing position.
4. *Toilet Hygiene*—Obtain and use supplies; clean self; transfer to and from, and maintain toileting position on, bedpan, toilet, or commode.
5. *Dressing*—Select appropriate clothing; obtain clothing from storage area; dress and

undress in a sequential fashion; and fasten and adjust clothing and shoes. Don and doff assistive or adaptive equipment, prostheses, or orthoses.

6. *Feeding and Eating*—Set up food; use appropriate utensils and tableware; bring food or drink to mouth; suck, masticate, cough, and swallow.
7. *Medication Routine*—Obtain medication; open and close containers; and take prescribed quantities as scheduled.
8. *Socialization*—Interact in appropriate contextual and cultural ways.
9. *Functional Communication*—Use equipment or systems to enhance or provide communication, such as writing equipment, telephones, typewriters, communication boards, call lights, emergency systems, braille writers, augmentative communication systems, and computers.
10. *Functional Mobility*—Move from one position or place to another, such as in bed mobility, wheelchair mobility, transfers (bed, car, tub, toilet, chair), and functional ambulation, with or without adaptive aids, driving, and use of public transportation.
11. *Sexual Expression*—Recognize, communicate, and perform desired sexual activities.

B. Work Activities

1. *Home Management*
   a. *Clothing Care*—Obtain and use supplies, launder, iron, store, and mend.
   b. *Cleaning*—Obtain and use supplies, pick up, vacuum, sweep, dust, scrub, mop, make bed, and remove trash.
   c. *Meal Preparation and Cleanup*—Plan nutritious meals and prepare food; open and close containers, cabinets, and drawers; use kitchen utensils and appliances; and clean up and store food.
   d. *Shopping*—Select and purchase items and perform money transactions.
   e. *Money Management*—Budget, pay bills, and use bank systems.
   f. *Household Maintenance*—Maintain home, yard, garden appliances, and household items, and/or obtain appropriate assistance.
   g. *Safety Procedures*—Know and perform prevention and emergency procedures to maintain a safe environment and prevent injuries.
2. *Care of Others*—Provide for children, spouse, parents, or others, such as the physical care, nurturance, communication, and use of age-appropriate activities.
3. *Educational Activities*—Participate in a school environment and school-sponsored activities (such as field trips, work-study, and extracurricular activities).
4. *Vocational Activities*
   a. *Vocational Exploration*—Determine aptitudes, interests, skills, and appropriate vocational pursuits.
   b. *Job Acquisition*—Identify and select work opportunities and complete application and interview processes.
   c. *Work or Job Performance*—Perform job tasks in a timely and effective manner, incorporating necessary work behaviors such as grooming, interpersonal skills, punctuality, and adherence to safety procedures.
   d. *Retirement Planning*—Determine aptitudes, interests, skills, and identify appropriate avocational pursuits.

C. Play or Leisure Activities

1. *Play or Leisure Exploration*—Identify interests, skills, opportunities, and appropriate play or leisure activities.
2. *Play or Leisure Performance*—Participate in play or leisure activities, using physical and psychosocial skills.
   a. Maintain a balance of play or leisure activities with work and activities of daily living.

b. Obtain, utilize, and maintain equipment and supplies.

II. PERFORMANCE COMPONENTS

A. Sensory Motor Component

1. *Sensory Integration*
   a. *Sensory Awareness*—Receive and differentiate sensory stimuli.
   b. *Sensory Processing*—Interpret sensory stimuli.
      (1) *Tactile*—Interpret light touch, pressure, temperature, pain, vibration, and two-point stimuli through skin contact/receptors.
      (2) *Proprioceptive*—Interpret stimuli originating in muscles, joints, and other internal tissues to give information about the position of one body part in relationship to another.
      (3) *Vestibular*—Interpret stimuli from the inner ear receptors regarding head position and movement.
      (4) *Visual*—Interpret stimuli through the eyes, including peripheral vision and acuity, awareness of color, depth, and figure-ground.
      (5) *Auditory*—Interpret sounds, localize sounds, and discriminate background sounds.
      (6) *Gustatory*—Interpret tastes.
      (7) *Olfactory*—Interpret odors.
   c. *Perceptual Skills*
      (1) *Stereognosis*—Identify objects through the sense of touch.
      (2) *Kinesthesia*—Identify the excursion and direction of joint movement.
      (3) *Body Scheme*—Acquire an internal awareness of the body and the relationship of body parts to each other.
      (4) *Right-Left Discrimination*—Differentiate one side of the body from the other.
      (5) *Form Constancy*—Recognize forms and objects as the same in various environments, positions, and sizes.
      (6) *Position in Space*—Determine the spatial relationship of figures and objects to self or other forms and objects.
      (7) *Visual Closure*—Identify forms or objects from incomplete presentations.
      (8) *Figure-Ground*—Differentiate between foreground and background forms and objects.
      (9) *Depth Perception*—Determine the relative distance between objects, figures, or landmarks and the observer.
      (10) *Topographical Orientation*—Determine the location of objects and settings and the route to the location.
2. *Neuromuscular*
   a. *Reflex*—Present an involuntary muscle response elicited by sensory input.
   b. *Range of Motion*—Move body parts through an arc.
   c. *Muscle Tone*—Demonstrate a degree of tension or resistance in a muscle.
   d. *Strength*—Demonstrate a degree of muscle power when movement is resisted as with weight or gravity.
   e. *Endurance*—Sustain cardiac, pulmonary, and musculoskeletal exertion over time.
   f. *Postural Control*—Position and maintain head, neck, trunk, and limb alignment with appropriate weight shifting, midline orientation, and righting reactions for function.
   g. *Soft Tissue Integrity*—Maintain anatomical and physiological condition of interstitial tissue and skin.
3. *Motor*
   a. *Activity Tolerance*—Sustain a purposeful activity over time.

b. *Gross Motor Coordination*—Use large muscle groups for controlled movements.
c. *Crossing the Midline*—Move limbs and eyes across the sagittal plane of the body.
d. *Laterality*—Use a preferred unilateral body part for activities requiring a high level of skill.
e. *Bilateral Integration*—Interact with both body sides in a coordinated manner during activity.
f. *Praxis*—Conceive and plan a new motor act in response to an environmental demand.
g. *Fine Motor Coordination/Dexterity*—Use small muscle groups for controlled movements, particularly in object manipulation.
h. *Visual-Motor Integration*—Coordinate the interaction of visual information with body movement during activity.
i. *Oral-Motor Control*—Coordinate oropharyngeal musculature for controlled movements.

B. Cognitive Integration and Cognitive Components
1. *Level of Arousal*—Demonstrate alertness and responsiveness to environmental stimuli.
2. *Orientation*—Identify person, place, time, and situation.
3. *Recognition*—Identify familiar faces, objects, and other previously presented materials.
4. *Attention Span*—Focus on a task over time.
5. *Memory*
   a. *Short-Term*—Recall information for brief periods of time.
   b. *Long-Term*—Recall information for long periods of time.
   c. *Remote*—Recall events from distant past.
   d. *Recent*—Recall events from immediate past.
6. *Sequencing*—Place information, concepts, and actions in order.
7. *Categorization*—Identify similarities of and differences between environmental information.
8. *Concept Formation*—Organize a variety of information to form thoughts and ideas.
9. *Intellectual Operations in Space*—Mentally manipulate spatial relationships.
10. *Problem Solving*—Recognize a problem, define a problem, identify alternative plans, select a plan, organize steps in a plan, implement a plan, and evaluate the outcome.
11. *Generalization of Learning*—Apply previously learned concepts and behaviors to similar situations.
12. *Integration of Learning*—Incorporate previously acquired concepts and behavior into a variety of new situations.
13. *Synthesis of Learning*—Restructure previously learned concepts and behaviors into new patterns.

C. Psychosocial Skills and Psychological Components
1. *Psychological*
   a. *Roles*—Identify functions one assumes or acquires in society (e.g., worker, student, parent, church member).
   b. *Values*—Identify ideas or beliefs that are intrinsically important.
   c. *Interests*—Identify mental or physical activities that create pleasure and maintain attention.
   d. *Initiation of Activity*—Engage in a physical or mental activity.
   e. *Termination of Activity*—Stop an activity at an appropriate time.
   f. *Self-Concept*—Develop value of physical and emotional self.

2. *Social*
   a. *Social Conduct*—Interact using manners, personal space, eye contact, gestures, active listening, and self-expression appropriate to one's environment.
   b. *Conversation*—Use verbal and non-verbal communication to interact in a variety of settings.
   c. *Self-Expression*—Use a variety of styles and skills to express thoughts, feelings, and needs.
3. *Self-Management*
   a. *Coping Skills*—Identify and manage stress and related reactors.
   b. *Time Management*—Plan and participate in a balance of self-care, work, leisure, and rest activities to promote satisfaction and health.
   c. *Self-Control*—Modulate and modify one's own behavior in response to environmental needs, demands, and constraints.

American Occupational Therapy Association, Inc.
Approved by the Representative Assembly April 1989

APPENDIX II

THE OCCUPATIONAL THERAPY WORKFORCE: 1989*

	OTRs Number	OTRs Percent	COTAs Number	COTAs Percent
U.S. Total	37600	100.00	9300	100.00
Alabama	290	0.77	104	1.12
Alaska	94	0.25	8	0.09
Arizona	470	1.25	56	0.60
Arkansas	196	0.52	7	0.08
California	4602	12.24	480	5.16
Colorado	978	2.60	84	0.90
Connecticut	643	1.71	192	2.06
Delaware	71	0.19	13	0.14
Dist. of Col.	98	0.26	8	0.09
Florida	1342	3.57	212	2.28
Georgia	534	1.42	43	0.46
Hawaii	256	0.68	73	0.79
Idaho	102	0.27	13	0.14
Illinois	1609	4.28	472	5.08
Indiana	654	1.74	159	1.71
Iowa	248	0.66	129	1.39
Kansas	549	1.46	87	0.94
Kentucky	207	0.55	25	0.27
Louisiana	425	1.13	47	0.50
Maine	263	0.70	39	0.42
Maryland	895	2.38	104	1.12
Massachusetts	1918	5.10	495	5.32
Michigan	2162	5.75	441	4.74
Minnesota	1402	3.73	864	9.29
Mississippi	83	0.22	12	0.13
Missouri	752	2.00	116	1.25
Montana	102	0.27	11	0.12
Nebraska	154	0.41	20	0.22
Nevada	83	0.22	12	0.13
New Hampshire	387	1.03	91	0.98
New Jersey	1049	2.79	187	2.01
New Mexico	241	0.64	17	0.18
New York	3290	8.75	1447	15.56
North Carolina	530	1.41	87	0.94
North Dakota	169	0.45	109	1.17
Ohio	1459	3.88	508	5.46

THE OCCUPATIONAL THERAPY WORKFORCE: 1989*
(continued)

Oklahoma	282	0.75	83	0.89
Oregon	447	1.19	119	1.28
Pennsylvania	1733	4.61	695	7.47
Puerto Rico	203	0.54	5	0.05
Rhode Island	132	0.35	17	0.18
South Carolina	233	0.62	23	0.25
South Dakota	79	0.21	20	0.22
Tennessee	278	0.74	135	1.45
Texas	1794	4.77	339	3.65
Utah	128	0.34	5	0.05
Vermont	83	0.22	21	0.23
Virginia	887	2.36	76	0.82
Virgin Islands	8	0.02	0	0.00
Washington	1154	3.07	189	2.03
West Virginia	53	0.14	8	0.09
Wisconsin	1737	4.62	787	8.46
Wyoming	64	0.17	4	0.04

*Estimates based on members and non-members of the AOTA.

Source: American Occupational Therapy Association Research Information and Evaluation Division.

APPENDIX III

OCCUPATIONAL THERAPY PERSONNEL CLASSIFICATIONS

CLASSIFICATION: STAFF CERTIFIED OCCUPATIONAL THERAPY ASSISTANT (COTA) ENTRY LEVEL

PRIMARY FUNCTION

To implement occupational therapy services for patients and clients under the supervision of an occupational therapist (OTR). These services include structured assessments, treatment, and documentation.

QUALIFICATIONS

1. Education: Graduate of an AOTA-approved occupational therapy assistant education program; successful completion of a minimum of two months supervised Level II Fieldwork experience; successful completion of the certification process for Occupational Therapy Assistant.
2. Certification and Licensure: Current AOTA certification; licensed as an Occupational Therapy Assistant where required by state law.
3. Experience: Less than one year of practice experience as a COTA.
4. Skills: Competent in the delivery of occupational therapy treatment, under the direction of an OTR as delineated in the AOTA Entry-Role Delineation for OTRs and COTAs.

EXAMPLES OF CRITICAL PERFORMANCE AREAS

- Indicates basic critical performance areas.
- Indicates performance areas at higher levels.

- Responds to requests for service by relaying information and referral to an OTR.
- Determines patient's/client's need for services in collaboration with an OTR.
- Contributes to the assessment process under supervision of an OTR.
- Assists OTR in developing treatment plans and techniques to implement plans.
- Monitors patient's/client's response to treatment and modifies treatment during sessions as indicated in collaboration with an OTR.
- Reports observations of patient's/client's performance and responses to services to the OTR.
- Recommends termination of patient/client services to the supervisor.
- Documents and maintains service-related records, as directed by supervising OTR.
- Assists in providing inservice education.
- Complies with established agency and service standards.
- Identifies own continuing education needs in consultation with OTR.

SUPERVISORY SUPPORT NEEDED

1. Clinical: Close supervision (i.e., daily direct contact on-site) is required from an OTR or intermediate or advanced level COTA.
2. Management/Administrative: General supervision by an experienced OTR or an experienced COTA is required for implementation of policies and procedures related to delivery of occupational therapy services.

CLASSIFICATION: STAFF CERTIFIED OCCUPATIONAL THERAPY ASSISTANT (COTA) INTERMEDIATE

PRIMARY FUNCTION

To implement occupational therapy services for patients/clients under the supervision of an occupational therapist (OTR). These services include structured evaluations, treatment, and documentation.

QUALIFICATIONS

1. Education: Graduate of an AOTA-approved occupational therapy assistant education program; successful completion of a minimum of two months supervised Level II Fieldwork experience; successful completion of the certification process for Occupational Therapy Assistant.
2. Certification and Licensure: Current AOTA certification; licensed as an Occupational Therapy Assistant where required by state law.
3. Experience: One or more years of practice as a COTA.
4. Skills: Competent in delivery of occupational therapy treatment under the direction of an OTR as delineated in the AOTA Entry-Level Role Delineation document; skill in implementation of a variety of independent living skills and activities that can be used in treatment; may be developing advanced-level skills in areas of special interest.

EXAMPLES OF CRITICAL PERFORMANCE AREAS

- Indicates basic critical performance areas.
- Indicates performance areas at higher levels.

- Responds to requests for service by relaying information and referral to an OTR.
- Determines patient's/client's need for services in collaboration with an OTR.
- Contributes to the patient's/client's assessment under supervision of an OTR. Independently performs parts of assessments, using structured evaluations.
- Assists OTR in developing treatment plans and techniques to implement plans.
- Implements and modifies treatment plans, under OTR supervision.
- Monitors patient's/client's response to treatment and modifies treatment during sessions, as indicated, in collaboration with OTR.
- Reports observations and patient's/client's responses to service to OTR and to other team members when so directed by OTR.
- Recommends to supervisor the termination of services.
- Documents and maintains service-related records, as directed by supervising OTR.
- Assists in the development of treatment protocols.
- Assists in the development of service records and procedures.
- Identifies own continuing education needs.
- Provides inservice education, and community education within scope of knowledge base.
- Provides administrative supervision and clinical direction to entry-level COTAs.
- Supervises OT aides and volunteers.
- Provides administration and clinical direction to OT Assistant Levels I and II fieldwork students.
- Assists OTR in the implementation of quality assurance program.
- Complies with established agency and service standards.

SUPERVISORY SUPPORT NEEDED

1. Clinical: General supervision (i.e., less than daily) from an intermediate or advanced level OTR is required. For COTAs with less than two years experience, close supervision (i.e., daily direct contact on-site) is preferred. The nature and frequency of supervision varies with patient/client populations. COTAs working with acutely ill patients/clients and with individuals who are making rapid changes will require more OTR supervision, due to the need for frequent

evaluation and re-evaluation and the resulting modification of overall treatment plan. COTAs treating patients/clients whose conditions are less complex and more stable, and therefore require program revisions less frequently, may be directed by the OTR to function more independently. Frequency and manner of contact is determined by the supervising OTR with on-site contact occurring at least monthly.

2. Management/Administrative: General supervision by an OTR experienced in administration or an advanced level COTA is required for implementation of policies and procedures related to the delivery of occupational therapy services.

CLASSIFICATION: STAFF CERTIFIED OCCUPATIONAL THERAPY ASSISTANT (COTA) ADVANCED

PRIMARY FUNCTION

An advanced level certified occupational therapy assistant (COTA) functioning as a staff member, but at a higher level than an intermediate COTA. Because of the variety of ways an individual may obtain advanced level skills and the variety of jobs that an individual may perform, specific qualifications and critical performance areas cannot be delineated. An advanced level COTA should be able to meet all the expectations of a STAFF COTA, INTERMEDIATE LEVEL, and the following education, experience, and skills.

QUALIFICATIONS

1. Education: Academic course work related to area of expertise from an accredited college or university; and/or certification related to a special area of practice by an organization or group that has continuing education, examination, and/or practice requirements; and/or extensive continuing education in special area of practice.
2. Experience: Three years or more experience in special area of practice.
3. Skills: A COTA in this category has advanced level competencies in particular acquired skills that relate to the practice of occupational therapy. These skills may be in clinically specific areas or may be more administrative or educational in nature. The advanced level COTA could be expected to share knowledge through staff and student education, publications, and clinical studies.

EXAMPLES OF CRITICAL PERFORMANCE AREAS

- Indicates basic critical performance areas.
- Because of the variety of ways an individual may obtain advanced level skills and the variety of jobs an individual may perform, critical performance areas at higher levels cannot be delineated.

- Responds to requests for service by relaying information and referral to an OTR.
- Determines patient's/client's need for services in collaboration with an OTR.
- Contributes to the patient's/client's assessment under supervision of an OTR. Independently performs parts of assessments, using structured evaluations.
- Assists OTR in developing treatment plans and techniques to implement plans.
- Implements and modifies treatment plans, under OTR supervision.
- Monitors patient's/client's response to treatment and modifies treatment during sessions, as indicated, in collaboration with OTR.
- Reports observations and patient's/client's responses to service to OTR and to other team members when so directed by OTR.
- Recommends to supervisor the termination of services.
- Documents and maintains service-related records, as directed by supervising OTR.
- Assists in the development of treatment protocols.

- Assists in the development of service records and procedures.
- Identifies own continuing education needs.
- Provides inservice education, and community education within scope of knowledge base.
- Provides administrative supervision and clinical direction to entry-level COTAs.
- Supervises OT aides and volunteers.
- Provides administration and clinical direction to OT Assistant Levels I and II fieldwork students.
- Assists OTR in the implementation of quality assurance program.
- Complies with established agency and service standards.

SUPERVISORY SUPPORT NEEDED

1. Clinical: General supervision (i.e., less than daily) from an intermediate or advanced-level OTR is required. The nature and frequency of supervision varies with patient's/client's population. COTAs working with acutely ill patients and with individuals who are making rapid changes will require more OTR supervision, because of the need for frequent evaluation and re-evaluation and resulting modification of overall treatment plan. COTAs treating patients whose conditions are less complex and more stable, therefore require program revisions less frequently, may be directed by the OTR to function more independently.
2. Management/Administrative: General supervision by an administratively experienced OTR is required for implementation of service policies and procedures.

Source: *COTA Supervision Guide*, Practice Division, American Occupational Therapy Association, 1986.

APPENDIX IV

TECHNICAL PROGRAMS 1989–1990

The following programs are approved by the American Occupational Therapy Association. On-site evaluations for program approval are conducted at 5-year intervals for initial approval and 7-year intervals for continuing approval. The dates on this list indicate the academic year the next evaluation is anticipated. For specific information, contact the program directly.

Key

1 Associate degree program
2 Certificate program
a Public
b Private nonprofit

ALABAMA

1, 2, a 89/90
University of Alabama at Birmingham
School of Health Related Professions
SHRP, Room 114
UAB Station
Birmingham, AL 35294
Carroline Amari, MA, OTR, Director
Occupational Therapy Assistant Program

CALIFORNIA

1, b 93/94
Loma Linda University
School of Allied Health Professions
Loma Linda, CA 92350
Lynn Arrateig, MA, OTR, Director
Occupational Therapy Assistant Program

COLORADO

1, a 90/91
Pueblo Community College
900 West Orman Avenue
Pueblo, CO 81004
Terry R. Hawkins, MPH, OTR, Chair
Occupational Therapy Assistant Program

CONNECTICUT

1, a 91/92
Manchester Community College
PO Box 1046, MS #19
Manchester, CT 06040
Brenda Smaga, MS, OTR/L, Coordinator
Occupational Therapy Assistant Program

FLORIDA

1, a 93/94
Palm Beach Community College
4200 Congress Avenue
Lake Worth, FL 33461
Sylvia Meeker, MS, OTR, Director
Occupational Therapy Assistant Program

GEORGIA

1, a 91/92
Medical College of Georgia
School of Allied Health Sciences
Augusta, GA 30912
Nancy Prendergast, EdD, OTR/L, FAOTA, Chair
Occupational Therapy Assistant Program

HAWAII

1, a **92/93**
University of Hawaii/Kapiolani Community College
Allied Health Department
4303 Diamond Head Road
Honolulu, HI 96816
Ann Kadoguchi, OTR, Director
Occupational Therapy Assistant Program

ILLINOIS

1, a **92/93**
Chicago City-Wide College/Cook County Hospital
Health Services Institute at Cook County Hospital
1900 West Polk Street
Chicago, IL 60612
Susan Kennedy, MS, OTR/L, Director
Occupational Therapy Assistant Program

1, a **92/93**
College of DuPage
Occupational and Vocational Education
22nd Street and Lambert Road
Glen Ellyn, IL 60137
Kathleen Mital, MOT, OTR, Director
Occupational Therapy Assistant Program

1, a **93/94**
Illinois Central College
East Peoria, IL 61635
Barbara J. Loar, MA, OTR/L, FAOTA, Acting Supervisor
Occupational Therapy Assistant Program
•Does not accept out-of-state students

1, a **91/92**
Parkland College
2400 West Bradley Avenue
Champaign, IL 61821–1899
Carol Ruch, OTR/L, Program Director
Occupational Therapy Assistant Program

1, a **90/91**
South Suburban College of Cook County
15800 South State Street
South Holland, IL 60473
Carolyn A. Yoss, OTR/L, Coordinator
Occupational Therapy Assistant Program

INDIANA

1*, a **95/96**
Indiana University School of Medicine
Division of Allied Health Sciences
1140 West Michigan Street CF 311
Indianapolis, IN 46202–5119
Celestine Hamant, MS, OTR, FAOTA, Associate Professor and Director
Occupational Therapy Assistant Program
•Admission to this program is closed

IOWA

1, a **89/90**
Kirkwood Community College
PO Box 2068
6301 Kirkwood Boulevard
Cedar Rapids, IA 52406
Mary Ellen Dunford, OTR/L, Director
Occupational Therapy Assistant Program

KANSAS

1, 2, a **91/92**
Barton County Community College
Great Bend, KS 67530
Program Director
Occupational Therapy Assistant Program

LOUISIANA

1, a **94/95**
Northeast Louisiana University
School of Allied Health Sciences
College of Pharmacy and Health Sciences
Monroe, LA 71209
Lee Sens, MA, OTR, Director
Occupational Therapy Assistant Program

MARYLAND

1, a **91/92**
Catonsville Community College
800 South Rolling Road
Baltimore, MD 21228
Judith Davis, MS, OTR, Coordinator
Occupational Therapy Assistant Program

MASSACHUSETTS

1, b **89/90**
Becker Junior College
61 Sever Street
Worcester, MA 01609
Edith C. Fenton, MS, OTR/L, Coordinator
Occupational Therapy Assistant Program

1, b 91/92
Mount Ida College
Junior College Division
777 Dedham Street
Newton Centre, MA 02159
Mira Coviensky, MS, OTR/L, Director
Occupational Therapy Assistant Program

1, a 94/95
North Shore Community College
3 Essex Street
Beverly, MA 01915
Sophia K. Fowler, MS, OTR/L, Director
Occupational Therapy Assistant Program

1, 2, a 91/92
Quinsigamond Community College
670 West Boylston Street
Worcester, MA 01606
Elaine Fallon, MS, OTR, FAOTA, Coordinator
Occupational Therapy Assistant Program

MICHIGAN

1, a 92/93
Grand Rapids Junior College
143 Bostwick, NE
Grand Rapids, MI 49503
Alice A. Donahue, MA, OTR, Director
Occupational Therapy Assistant Program

1, a 91/92
Schoolcraft College
1751 Radcliff Street
Garden City, MI 48135-1197
Masline Horton, MS, EdSp, OTR,
Professor/Coordinator
Occupational Therapy Assistant Program

1, a 94/95
Wayne County Community College
1001 West Fort Street
Detroit, MI 48226
Doris Y. Witherspoon, MA, OTR, Director
Occupational Therapy Assistant Program

MINNESOTA

1, a 89/90
Anoka Technical Institute*
1355 West Highway 10
Anoka, MN 55303
Marcia S. Urseth, OTR, Program Chair
Occupational Therapy Assistant Program
*In cooperation with Anoka Ramsey Community College

1, a 92/93
Austin Community College
1600 8th Avenue, NW
Austin, MN 55912
Thomas H. Dillon, MA, OTR,
Program Director
Occupational Therapy Assistant Program
Offered: Austin, Worthington*
*Pending approval

1, a 92/93
Duluth Technical Institute*
2101 Trinity Road
Duluth, MN 55811
Julie A. Halom, OTR, Director
Occupational Therapy Assistant Program
*In cooperation with Hibbing Community College

1, b 92/93
St. Mary's Campus of the College of St. Catherine
2500 South Sixth Street
Minneapolis, MN 55454
Marianne F. Christiansen, MA, OTR, Director
Occupational Therapy Assistant Program

MISSOURI

1, a 90/91
Penn Valley Community College
3201 Southwest Trafficway
Kansas City, MO 64111
Janice S. Bacon, OTR, Program Coordinator
Occupational Therapy Assistant Program

1, a 89/90
St. Louis Community College at Meramec
11333 Big Bend Boulevard
St. Louis, MO 63122
Lee Frye, MS, OTR, Director
Occupational Therapy Assistant Program

NEW HAMPSHIRE

1, a 95/96
New Hampshire Technical College–Claremont
One College Drive
Claremont, NH 03743-9707
Joan Holcombe Larsen, MEd, OTR, Director
Occupational Therapy Assistant Program

NEW JERSEY

1, a 95/96
Atlantic Community College
Allied Health Division
Mays Landing, NJ 08330
Angela J. Busillo, MEd, OTR, Director
Occupational Therapy Assistant Program

1, a 93/94
Union County College
1700 Raritan Road
Scotch Plains, NJ 07076
Carol Keating, MA, OTR, Program Director
Occupational Therapy Assistant Program

NEW YORK

1, a 95/96
Erie Community College
Main Street and Youngs Road
Buffalo, NY 14221
Sally Jo Harris, MS, OTR/L, Director
Occupational Therapy Assistant Program

1, a 93/94
Herkimer County Community College
Herkimer, NY 13350
Brice Kistler, OTR/L, Program Director
Occupational Therapy Assistant Program

1, a 90/91
LaGuardia Community College
31-10 Thomson Avenue
Long Island City, NY 11101
Naomi Greenberg, MPH, PhD, OTR, FAOTA, Director
Occupational Therapy Assistant Program

1, b 92/93
Maria College
700 New Scotland Avenue
Albany, NY 12208
Sandra C. Jung, OTR, Program Chair
Occupational Therapy Assistant Program

1*, b 94/95
Maria Regina College
Allied Health Division
1024 Court Street
Syracuse, NY 13208
Sr. Thomas Marie Corcoran, MS, OTR, Director
Occupational Therapy Assistant Program
*Admission to this program is closed

1, a 95/96
Orange County Community College
115 South Street
Middletown, NY 10940
Mary Sands, MSEd, OTR, Chair
Occupational Therapy Assistant Program

1, a 92/93
Rockland Community College
145 College Road
Suffern, NY 10901
Ellen Spergel, MS, OTR, Director
Occupational Therapy Assistant Program

NORTH CAROLINA

1, a 95/96
Caldwell Community College and Technical Institute
1000 Hickory Boulevard
Hudson, NC 28638
Lyndon Lackey, OTR/L, Coordinator
Occupational Therapy Assistant Program

1, a 94/95
Stanly Community College
Route 4, Box 55
Albemarle, NC 28001
Nancy Glover, MS, OTR/L, Director
Occupational Therapy Assistant Program

NORTH DAKOTA

1, a 93/94
North Dakota State College of Science
Wahpeton, ND 58075
Sr. Carolita Mauer, MA, OTR/L, Chair
Occupational Therapy Assistant Program

OHIO

1, a 92/93
Cincinnati Technical College
3520 Central Parkway
Cincinnati, OH 45223
Sandra Driskell Prantl, OTR, Program Director
Occupational Therapy Assistant Program

1, a 94/95
Cuyahoga Community College
2900 Community College Avenue
Cleveland, OH 44115
Debbra H. Lisy, MA, OTR/L, Acting Program Manager
Occupational Therapy Assistant Program

1, b 90/91
Lourdes College
6832 Convent Boulevard
Sylvania, OH 43560
Cynthia Goodwin, OTR/L, Director
Occupational Therapy Assistant Program

1, a 90/91
Shawnee State University
940 Second Street
Portsmouth, OH 45662
Program Director
Occupational Therapy Assistant Program

1, a 89/90
Stark Technical College
6200 Frank Avenue, NW
Canton, OH 44720
Johannes Kicken, MS, OTR, Director
Occupational Therapy Assistant Program

OKLAHOMA

1, a 94/95
Oklahoma City Community College
7777 South May Avenue
Oklahoma City, OK 73159
Margaret F. Roseboom, OTR, Coordinator
Occupational Therapy Assistant Program

OREGON

1, a 95/96
Mount Hood Community College
26000 SE Stark Street
Gresham, OR 97030
Chris Hencinski, OTR, Coordinator
Occupational Therapy Assistant Program

PENNSYLVANIA

1, a 89/90
Community College of Allegheny County
Boyce Campus
595 Beatty Road
Monroeville, PA 15146
Richard L. Allison, MS, OTR/L, Director
Occupational Therapy Assistant Program

1, b 91/92
Harcum Junior College
Bryn Mawr, PA 19010
Jerald P. Stowell, MPH, OTR, Director
Occupational Therapy Assistant Program

1, a 94/95
Lehigh County Community College
2370 Main Street
Schnecksville, PA 18078
Dorothy J. Grabowski, OTR/L, Coordinator
Occupational Therapy Assistant Program

1, b 91/92
Mount Aloysius Junior College
Cresson, PA 16630
M. Teresa Moler, MA, OTR/L, Acting Chair
Occupational Therapy Assistant Program

1, a 92/93
Pennsylvania College of Technology
One College Avenue
Williamsport, PA 17701-5799
Barbara N. Sims, OTR/L,
Program Coordinator
Occupational Therapy Assistant Program

PUERTO RICO

1, a 89/90
Humacao University College
CUH Postal Station
Humacao, PR 00661
Dyhalma Irizarry, PhD, OTR,
Program Director
Occupational Therapy Assistant Program

1, a 91/92
Ponce Technological University College
University of Puerto Rico
PO Box 7186
Ponce, PR 00732
Ana V. Ferran, PhD, OTR, Coordinator
Occupational Therapy Assistant Program

SOUTH CAROLINA

1, a 93/94
Trident Technical College
PO Box 10367
Charleston, SC 29411
Penny Pratt, MHE, OTR, Director
Occupational Therapy Assistant Program

TENNESSEE

1, a 92/93
Nashville State Technical Institute
120 White Bridge Road
PO Box 90285
Nashville, TN 37209
Anne K. Brown, MS, OTR, Program Director
Occupational Therapy Assistant Program

TEXAS

2, a 92/93
Academy of Health Sciences, U.S. Army
Medicine & Surgery Division
Fort Sam Houston, TX 78234-6100
LTC Wade W. Daigle, PhD, OTR, Chief
Occupational Therapy Branch
Occupational Therapy Assistant Program
(Limited to enlisted personnel in Army and Air Force)

1, a 89/90
Austin Community College
Riverside Campus
5712 East Riverside Drive
Austin, TX 78741
Martha Sue Carrell, OTR, Department Head
Occupational Therapy Assistant Program

2, a 93/94
Houston Community College
3100 Shenandoah
Houston, TX 77021
Linda Williams, MA, OTR, Coordinator
Occupational Therapy Assistant Program

1, a 90/91
St. Philip's College
2111 Nevada Street
San Antonio, TX 78203
Jana Cragg, OTR, Program Director
Occupational Therapy Assistant Program

WASHINGTON

1, a 89/90
Green River Community College
12401 SE 320th Street
Auburn, WA 98002
Barbara J. Rom, MS, OTR/L, Program Coordinator
Occupational Therapy Assistant Program

1, a 93/94
Yakima Valley Community College
Sixteenth Avenue and Nob Hill Boulevard
PO Box 1647
Yakima, WA 98907
Peg Bryant, OTR/L, Program Director
Occupational Therapy Assistant Program

WISCONSIN

1, a 93/94
Fox Valley Technical College
1825 North Bluemound Drive
PO Box 2277
Appleton, WI 54913
Patricia Holz, OTR, Coordinator
Occupational Therapy Assistant Program

1, a 95/96
Madison Area Technical College
211 North Carroll Street
Madison, WI 53703-2285
Toni Walski, MS, OTR, Director
Occupational Therapy Assistant Program

1, a 94/95
Milwaukee Area Technical College
700 West State Street
Milwaukee, WI 53233
Suzanne L. Brown, MS, OTR, Coordinator
Occupational Therapy Assistant Program

DEVELOPING TECHNICAL PROGRAMS 1989–1990

The following programs are in the developing stage and are not yet approved by the American Occupational Therapy Association. The dates of the academic year for the initial on-site evaluation of the program appear in the listing. For specific information, contact the program directly.

OHIO

1, a 89/90
Muskingum Area Technical College
1555 Newark Road
Zanesville, OH 43701
Karen Linser, OTR/L, Program Coordinator.
Occupational Therapy Assistant Program

1, a 90/91
Sinclair Community College
444 West Third Street
Dayton, OH 45402
S. Kay Ashworth, MAT, OTR/L, Chair
Occupational Therapy Assistant Program

PENNSYLVANIA

1, a 91/92
The Pennsylvania State University
University Park, PA 16802
Haru Hirama, EdD, OTR/L, Program Director
Occupational Therapy Assistant Program
Offered: Berks, Mont Alto only

CALIFORNIA

1, a 90/91
Sacramento City College
3835 Freeport Boulevard
Sacramento, CA 95822
Geri Liebert, MA, OTR, Coordinator
Occupational Therapy Assistant Program

1, a 89/90
San Jose City College
2100 Moorpark Avenue
San Jose, CA 95128–2799
Peg Bledsoe, MA, OTR, Acting Co-director
Peggy Owens, OTR, Acting Co-director
Occupational Therapy Assistant Program

MONTANA

2; a 90/91
Great Falls Vocational-Technical Center
2100 16th Avenue South
Great Falls, MT 59405
Judith Patrick, OTR, Program Director
Occupational Therapy Assistant Program

The American Journal of Occupational Therapy, 1989

APPENDIX V

CONTACTS FOR OCCUPATIONAL THERAPY REGULATORY BOARDS

The following list contains information about 37 states, the District of Columbia, and Puerto Rico with occupational therapy regulatory laws. Seven additional states (Arizona, Indiana, Michigan, Minnesota, Missouri, Virginia and Wisconsin) were regulated in 1988–1989.

Alaska
Enactment date: 1987
Direct requests to:
Wanda Flemming, Licensing Examiner
State of Alaska, Department of Commerce
Division of Occupational Licensing
State OT & PT Board
P.O. Box D-LIC
Juneau, AK 99811

Arkansas
Enactment date: 1977
Direct requests to:
Joe Verser, M.D.
Secretary/Treasurer
Arkansas State Medical Board
P.O. Box 102
Harrisburg, AR 72432
(501) 578-2677

Connecticut
Enactment date: 1979
Direct requests to:
Connecticut State Department
of Health Services
Division of Medical Quality Assurance
150 Washington Street
Hartford, CT 06106
(203) 566-1039

Delaware
Enactment date: 1985
Direct requests to:
Elizabeth Hutchins
DE State Board of OT
Division of Professional Regulation
Margaret O'Neill Bldg.
P.O. Box 1401
Dover, DE 19903

District of Columbia
Enactment date: 1978
Direct requests to:
Board of Occupational Therapy
Practice
Occupational and Professional
Licensing Administration
614 H Street, N.W., Room 923
Washington, D.C. 20001
(202) 727-7468

Florida
Enactment date: 1975
Amended: 1978
Direct requests to:
Department of Professional
Regulation
Florida Board of Medical
Examiners
130 North Monroe Street
Tallahassee, FL 32301
(904) 488-0595

*Please send a copy of all
information sent to the
Florida Licensure Board to:
Catherine Seidl
3301 SW 40th Avenue
Hollywood, FL 33023

Georgia
Enactment date: 1976
Direct requests to:
Georgia Board of Occupational
Therapy
Examining Board Division
166 Pryor Street, S.W.
Atlanta, GA 30303
(404) 656-3921

Idaho
Enactment date: 1987
Direct requests to:
Rhea Velasquez
Administrative Assistant
Idaho State Board of Medicine
500 S. 10th Street, Suite 103
State House
Boise, ID 83720

Illinois
Enactment date: 1983
Direct requests to:
Illinois Department of
Registration and Education
320 West Washington Street, 3rd Floor
Springfield, IL 62786
(217) 785-0800

Iowa
Enactment date: 1980
Direct requests to:
Iowa State Board of PT/OT Examiners
Professional Licensure
State Department of Health
Lucas State Office Building
Des Moines, IA 50319
(515) 281-4401

Kansas
Enactment date: 1986
Direct requests to:
Kansas State Board of Healing Arts
London State Office Bldg.
900 S.W. Jackson, Suite 553
Topeka, KS 66612

Kentucky
Enactment date: 1986
Direct requests to:
Kentucky Occupational Therapy
License Board
P.O. Box 23562
Lexington, KY 40523

Louisiana
Enactment date: 1979
Direct requests to:
Louisiana State Board of Medical Examiners
Occupational Therapy Division
830 Union Street, Suite 100
New Orleans, LA 70112
(504) 524-6763

Maine
Enactment date: 1984
Direct requests to:
Jean Blanchard
39 Foreside Common Drive
Falmouth, ME 04105
Work: (207) 871-2523

Maryland
Enactment date: 1978
Direct requests to:
Board of Occupational Therapy
Practice
Department of Health and
Mental Hygiene
O'Conor State Office Building
201 West Preston Street
First Floor
Baltimore, MD 21201
(301) 383-7024

Massachusetts
Enactment date: 1983
Direct requests to:
Board of Registration in
Allied Health Professions
100 Cambridge Street
Room 1509
Boston, MA 02202
(617) 727-3076 ext. 61

Montana
Enactment date: April 1985
Direct requests to:
Debbie Ammondson
200 13th Avenue, South #23
Great Falls, MT 59405
Work: (406) 727-3333 ext. 5203

Nebraska
Enactment date: 1984
Direct requests to:
JoAnn Erickson
Associate Director
Bureau of Examining Boards
Department of Health
P.O. Box 95007
Lincoln, NE 68509
(402) 471-2115

New Hampshire
Enactment date: 1977
Direct requests to:
New Hampshire Board of
Registration in Medicine
Occupational Therapy Licensure
Health and Welfare Building
Hazen Drive
Concord, NH 03301
(603) 271-4502

New Mexico
Enactment date: 1983
Direct requests to:
New Mexico Board of
Occupational Therapy Practice
P.O. Box 35370
Albuquerque, NM 87176
(505) 281-1932

New York
Enactment date: 1975
Amended: 1977
Direct requests to:
Division of Professional
Licensing
Occupational Therapy Unit
Cultural Education Center
Madison Avenue
Albany, NY 12203
(518) 474-3833

North Carolina
Enactment date: 1984
Direct requests to:
Jane Rourk
808 Wells Street
Durham, NC 27707
Work: (919) 966-5796

North Dakota
Enactment date: 1983
Direct requests to:
State Board of Occupational
Therapy Practice
University Station
Box 8066
Grand Forks, ND 58202

Ohio
Enactment date: 1975
Direct requests to:
Ohio Occupational and Physical
Therapy Board
65 South Front Street
Room 217
Columbus, OH 43215
(614) 466-3774

Oklahoma
Enactment date: 1984
Direct requests to:
Board of Medical Examiners
Box 18256
Oklahoma City, OK 73154
(405) 842-5674

Oregon
Enactment date: 1977
Direct requests to:
Oregon State Board of
Occupational Therapy
1400 Southwest 5th Street
Portland, OR 97201
(503) 229-5160

Pennsylvania
Enactment date: 1982
Direct requests to:
State Board of Occupational Therapy
Education and Licensure
Box 2649
Harrisburg, PA 17105-2649
(717) 783-1400

Puerto Rico
Enactment date: 1968
Direct requests to:
Departamento De Salud
Junta Examinadora De
Terapia Ocupacional
Box 9342
Santurce, PR 00908

Rhode Island
Enactment date: 1984
Direct requests to:
Department of Health
Professional Regulation
75 Davis Street, Room 104
Providence, RI 02908
(401) 277-2827

South Dakota
Enactment date: 1986
Direct requests to:
SD Board of Medical Examiners
1323 S. Minnesota Ave.
Sioux Falls, SD 57105

Tennessee
Due to sunset review of the healing arts board, the effective date of the legislation has been delayed. No licenses are being issued at this time.
Enactment date: 1983
Direct requests to:
Mary Collier
2918 Hillsboro Road, Apt. L-3
Nashville, TN 37215
or
Kathy Pire
3600 Hillsboro Road, Apt. B-2
Nashville, TN 37215

Texas
Enactment date: 1983
Direct requests to:
Cary Westhouse, OTR
Executive Director of
Licensure Board
Texas Advisory Board for
Occupational Therapy
Texas Rehabilitation Commission
118 East Riverside Drive
Suite 243
Austin, TX 78704
(512) 445-8368

Utah
Enactment date: 1977
Direct requests to:
Utah State Occupational Therapy
Advisory Committee
Division of Registration
160 East 300, South
P.O. Box 5802
Salt Lake City, UT 84110
(801) 530-6633

Washington
Enactment date: February 1984
Direct requests to:
Cynthia Jones
Washington State
Licensure Board
Division of
Professional Licensing
P.O. Box 9649
Olympia, WA 98504
(206) 753-6936

West Virginia
Enactment date: 1978
Direct requests to:
Frances Ingram, Secretary
West Virginia Board of
Occupational Therapy
P.O. Box 384
Dunbar, WV 25064
Home: (304) 722-2640
Work: (304) 768-8861

California
A trademark bill was enacted in 1977 to protect the title "occupational therapy" and to prevent facilities from advertising occupational therapy unless they have a qualified therapist. The law stipulates that only people who meet the requirements for AOTA certification may represent themselves as occupational therapists or occupational therapy assistants. The law is enforced by the California Department of Health which is responsible for licensing all health facilities.
In 1983, a bill was introduced adding a scope of practice definition to the 1977 law as well as a statement protecting the practice of occupational therapy. This bill was not heard by committee and in 1984 a second bill will be introduced.

Hawaii

The Hawaii trademark law was enacted in May 1978. The law reserves the use of the title "Occupational Therapist" and "Occupational Therapy Assistant" (or OT, letters, abbreviations, or insignias) to only those individuals who have met the requirements for certification by The American Occupational Therapy Association.

Compiled by American Occupational Therapy Association, August 1989.

APPENDIX VI

OCCUPATIONAL THERAPY CODE OF ETHICS

The American Occupational Therapy Association and its component members are committed to furthering people's ability to function fully within their total environment. To this end the occupational therapist renders service to clients in all stages of health and illness, to institutions, to other professionals and colleagues, to students, and to the general public.

In furthering this commitment, the American Occupational Therapy Association has established the Occupational Therapy Code of Ethics. This code is intended to be used as a guide to promoting and maintaining the highest standards of ethical behavior.

This Code of Ethics shall apply to all occupational therapy personnel. The term *occupational therapy personnel* shall include individuals who are registered occupational therapists, certified occupational therapy assistants, and occupational therapy students. The roles of practitioner, educator, manager, researcher, and consultant are assumed.

Principle 1 (Beneficence/Autonomy)

Occupational therapy personnel shall demonstrate a concern for the welfare and dignity of the recipient of their services.

A. The individual is responsible for providing services without regard to race, creed, national origin, sex, age, handicap, disease entity, social status, financial status, or religious affiliation.
B. The individual shall inform those people served of the nature and potential outcomes of treatment and shall respect the right of potential recipients of service to refuse treatment.
C. The individual shall inform subjects involved in education or research activities of the potential outcome of those activities.
D. The individual shall include those people served in the treatment planning process.
E. The individual shall maintain goal-directed and objective relationships with all people served.
F. The individual shall protect the confidential nature of information gained from educational, practice, and investigational activities unless sharing such information could be deemed necessary to protect the well-being of a third party.
G. The individual shall take all reasonable precautions to avoid harm to the recipient of services or detriment to the recipient's property.
H. The individual shall establish fees, based on cost analysis, that are commensurate with services rendered.

Principle 2 (Competence)

Occupational therapy personnel shall actively maintain high standards of professional competence.

A. The individual shall hold the appropriate credential for providing service.
B. The individual shall recognize the need for competence and shall participate in continuing professional development.
C. The individual shall function within the parameters of his or her competence and the standards of the profession.

D. The individual shall refer clients to other service providers or consult with other service providers when additional knowledge and expertise is required.

Principle 3 (Compliance With Laws and Regulations)

Occupational therapy personnel shall comply with laws and Association policies guiding the profession of occupational therapy.

A. The individual shall be acquainted with applicable local, state, federal, and institutional rules and Association policies and shall function accordingly.
B. The individual shall inform employers, employees, and colleagues about those laws and policies that apply to the profession of occupational therapy.
C. The individual shall require those whom they supervise to adhere to the Code of Ethics.
D. The individual shall accurately record and report information.

Principle 4 (Public Information)

Occupational therapy personnel shall provide accurate information concerning occupational therapy services.

A. The individual shall accurately represent his or her competence and training.
B. The individual shall not use or participate in the use of any form of communication that contains a false, fraudulent, deceptive, or unfair statement or claim.

Principle 5 (Professional Relationships)

Occupational therapy personnel shall function with discretion and integrity in relations with colleagues and other professionals, and shall be concerned with the quality of their services.

A. The individual shall report illegal, incompetent, and/or unethical practice to the appropriate authority.
B. The individual shall not disclose privileged information when participating in reviews of peers, programs, or systems.
C. The individual who employs or supervises colleagues shall provide appropriate supervision, as defined in AOTA guidelines or state laws, regulations, and institutional policies.
D. The individual shall recognize the contributions of colleagues when disseminating professional information.

Principle 6 (Professional Conduct)

Occupational therapy personnel shall not engage in any form of conduct that constitutes a conflict of interest or that adversely reflects on the profession.

This document was approved by the Representative Assembly in April 1988; it replaces the (1977/1979) "Principles of Occupational Therapy Ethics."

American Occupational Therapy Association, 1988.

INDEX

I

J

K

L

M

N

O

P

Q

R

S

U

V

W

Y